30-SECOND
NUTRITION

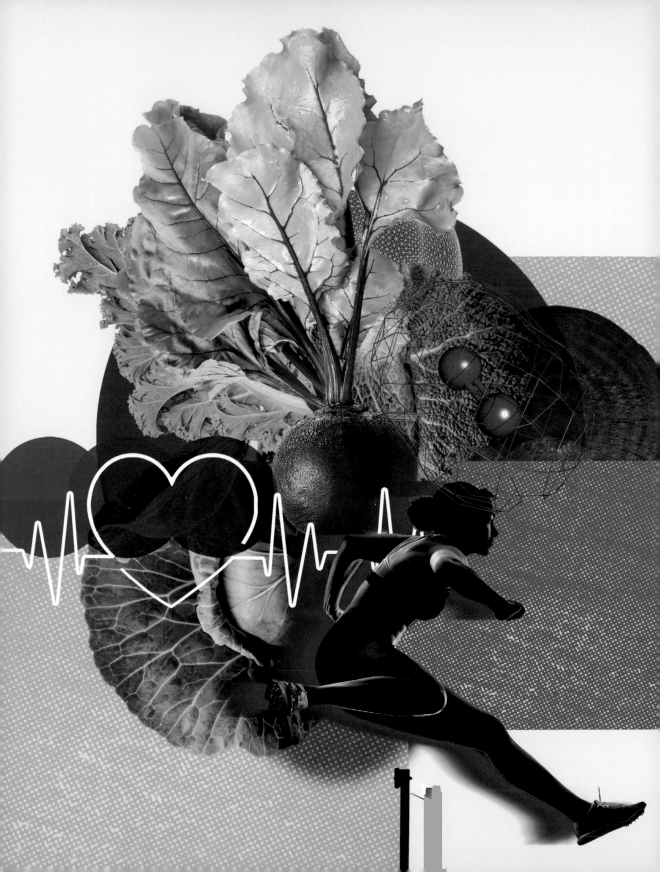

30-SECOND NUTRITION

The 50 most significant
nutrition-related facts, each
explained in half a minute

Editor
Julie A Lovegrove

Contributors
Margaret Ashwell
Luke Bell
Jenna Braddock
Philip C Calder
Rosalind Fallaize
Glenn Gibson
Ian Givens
Bruce A Griffin
Kristen Hicks-Roof
Ditte Hobbs
Ian Macdonald

Oonagh Markey
Elizabeth A Miles
D Joe Millward
Brian Power
Hilary Powers
Judith Rodriguez
Carrie Ruxton
Jill Snyder
Katherine Stephens
Jayne Woodside
Zhiping Yu

Illustrator
Steve Rawlings

IVY PRESS

First published in the UK in 2018 by
Ivy Press
An imprint of The Quarto Group
The Old Brewery, 6 Blundell Street
London N7 9BH, United Kingdom
T (0)20 7700 6700 **F** (0)20 7700 8066
www.QuartoKnows.com

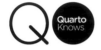

British Library Cataloguing-in-
Publication Data
A catalogue record for this
book is available from the
British Library.

ISBN: 978-1-78240-553-5

This book was conceived,
designed and produced by
Ivy Press
58 West Street, Brighton BN1 2RA, UK

Publisher **Susan Kelly**
Creative Director **Michael Whitehead**
Editorial Director **Tom Kitch**
Art Director **James Lawrence**
Project Editor **Katie Crous**
Designer **Ginny Zeal**

Printed in China

10 9 8 7 6 5 4 3 2 1

CONTENTS

INTRODUCTION
Julie Lovegrove

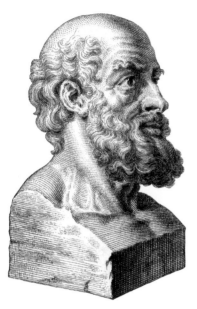

Hippocrates proposed that following a balanced diet and avoiding excessive consumption were important for good health.

Nutrition has been defined as 'the process of providing or obtaining food necessary for health and growth' (*Oxford Dictionary*), and is essential for sustaining all life on Earth. The word 'nutrition' originates from the sixteenth century, from late Latin *nūtrītiō*, 'to nourish'. The quality of our diet influences our development and well-being from the womb until death, and is, therefore, of relevance to all. Our instinct to eat is principally for survival, but the selection of foods is determined by the environment, genetics and numerous other factors. Understanding the principles of nutrition and how different foods and nutrients promote health and prevent disease empowers humans to make an informed choice, optimizing their diet.

The Greek physician Hippocrates of Kos (460–370 BCE), known as the 'Father of Medicine', was one of the first to profess the importance of nutrition, stating, 'Let food be thy medicine and medicine be thy food.' Hippocrates recognized the therapeutic significance of diet for the maintenance of health, and developed one of the earliest nutritional recommendations that he called a 'seasonal diet'. In the Tang dynasty (618–907 CE), Chinese physician Sun Simiao wrote what could be regarded to be the first nutrition guidelines in his book *Precious Prescriptions for Emergencies*, which described the impacts of consuming grains, meat, fruits and vegetables. It wasn't until the twentieth century that formal public health dietary recommendations came into effect for populations across the world.

A landmark discovery in the history of nutritional science occurred in the nineteenth century with the recognition of a causal link between malnourishment and disease, and the first description of essential micronutrients as 'vitamines' in 1912 by Casimir Funk. Following this, Frederick Hopkins, an English biochemist, was awarded the Nobel Prize in Physiology or Medicine for the discovery of the 'growth-stimulating vitamins' in 1929. The identification of vitamins was viewed by many as an endpoint to the study of nutrition, a short-sighted view given the significant developments that were to follow. The increasing prevalence of chronic degenerative diseases like heart disease and cancer as major causes of premature death in the Western world in the late twentieth century refocused attention on the importance of over-nutrition and the role of macronutrients in disease development.

Ongoing challenges in the field of nutritional science include: developing more definitive measures of dietary intake; health status; and disease risk susceptibility in the early stages of life, when nutrition can be more effective in maintaining health and preventing disease. These challenges are being tackled by the development of new analytical techniques, identification of novel biological markers of dietary intake and disease risk, and innovations in food science and technology. Progressions in nutritional science have occurred in parallel with advances in genetic, metabolic and behavioural sciences, that will continue to improve tailored dietary advice to specific characteristics of an individual to motivate changes in diet for health.

The aims of *30-Second Nutrition* are to provide insight into the fundamental importance of nutrition to life, and to increase understanding of the principles of nutrition, to help readers make informed decisions about their diet and food choice.

Sun Simiao advocated treatment of diseases through diet, in addition to specific herbal remedies.

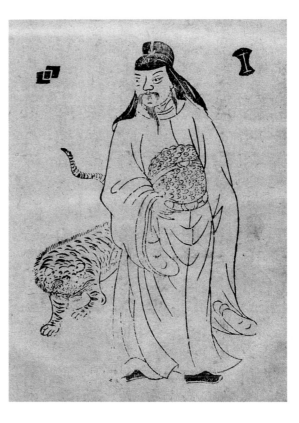

About this book

30-Second Nutrition is your bitesize guide to food and its nutrients: covering the science behind bodily functions that help us to digest and absorb; through food groups and their impact on health; to how food is grown and processed. Experts – nutritionists, dietitians, academics, researchers – from around the globe share their knowledge and guide us through the carefully selected topics, to ensure all fundamental bases are covered, clearly and concisely. The gen on each topic is presented on a single page, with an accompanying artwork on the opposite page to encapsulate its essence. The main paragraph, the 30-Second Digest, is complemented by the 3-Second Bite, which gives a quicker overview – the key facts in a single sentence. And the 3-Minute Snack fleshes this out, adding intriguing aspects of the subject. Each chapter also contains a biography of a pioneer in the field – the men and women who contributed to our understanding of modern nutrition. The book begins with an overview of the main groups of nutrients in food and how our bodies work to process and use these nutrients. It then delves into food groups and their related health benefits, or otherwise. As nutritional demands change through life, there is a chapter that takes you through the key stages of the life cycle. Then it's on to the potential hazards associated with some food groups and the various risks they can pose to health, but also looking at the ways in which we may be able to influence our diet and health more positively. The final chapter takes a modern-day look at food processing and production, helping us to evaluate the ever-widening range of food-related choices on offer.

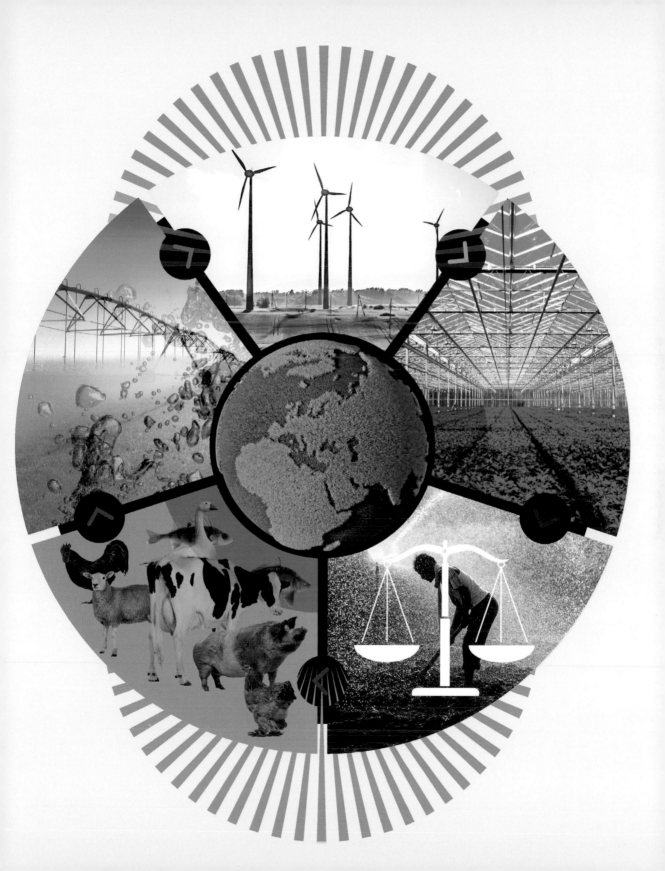

NUTRIENTS: LIFE'S ESSENTIALS

NUTRIENTS: LIFE'S ESSENTIALS
GLOSSARY

amino acids The building blocks of all proteins, amino acids make up a large proportion of cells, muscles and tissue, carrying out many important bodily functions, such as giving cells their structure. Also play a key role in the transport and storage of nutrients. Essential amino acids need to be gained through diet rather than formed by the body itself.

anaemia Develops when the blood does not contain enough healthy red blood cells or haemoglobin, important for carrying oxygen around the body. There are many types and causes, including iron deficiency. Symptoms include lethargy, shortness of breath, pale complexion and dry nails.

cell signalling The communication of cells by sending and receiving chemical signals, which allow the cells in your body to coordinate their activities, such as development, tissue repair and immunity. Errors in signalling contribute to diseases such as cancer, autoimmunity and diabetes.

disaccharides 'Double sugar' made of two molecules of **simple sugars** linked to each other. Include sucrose, maltose and lactose.

eicosanoids Compounds responsible for many of the beneficial effects of good fats; however, some are potentially harmful if excessive amounts build up in the body.

fatty acids The building blocks of fat in the body and in food. During digestion, the body breaks down fats into fatty acids, which can then be absorbed into the blood. Essential fatty acids (EFAs) must be ingested because the body requires them for good health but cannot synthesize them. Those not essential are non-essential fatty acids.

folate Also known as vitamin B_9. Folate in the form of folic acid is advised for pregnant women (to prevent neural tube defects in the developing foetus) and to prevent a type of **anaemia**. Essential for DNA synthesis and metabolizing amino acids, it is a dietary requirement – an essential vitamin.

free radicals Cells consist of molecules; molecules consist of atoms joined by chemical bonds. When a bond breaks, a free radical is formed, which can set off a degenerative process that damages the cell. Free radicals can be formed during metabolism, by the immune system as a response to illness, by the ageing process, or due to environmental factors such as pollution.

glycaemic index (GI) Rating system for foods containing carbohydrates, showing how quickly each food affects your blood sugar (glucose) level when consumed on its own. Carbohydrate-rich foods, including sugary foods and drinks, white bread and potatoes, have a high GI rating. Low GI foods include some fruit and vegetables, pulses and wholegrain foods. Low GI foods are generally considered more healthy than high GI foods, although foods with a high GI are not necessarily unhealthy and not all foods with a low GI are healthy.

macronutrients Three main components of the diet: fat, protein and carbohydrate. All have their own specific functions in the body, and all supply calories or energy. Required in relatively large amounts to grow, develop and thrive.

osteomalacia Rickets in adults; a softening of the bones caused by a lack of vitamin D or calcium. Symptoms include bone pain, difficulty in walking, easy fracturing of bones and a compressed vertebrae.

peptide bonds Covalent bond formed between two amino acids. Living organisms use bonds to form long chains of amino acids, known as proteins.

polysaccharides Carbohydrate (for example starch, cellulose and glycogen) whose molecules consist of a number of sugar molecules bonded together. Serve as short-term energy stores.

simple sugars Called 'monosaccharides'; made up of single sugar molecules. Include glucose and fructose. Present in natural and processed foods. See also **disaccharides**.

thiamin (vitamin B$_1$) Water-soluble vitamin that enables the body to use carbohydrates as energy. Essential for glucose metabolism; plays a key role in nerve, muscle and heart function.

total energy expenditure (TEE) Depends on the rate at which the body expends energy at rest (basal metabolic rate – BMR) and our physical activity level (PAL), and this is expressed by the relationship: TEE = PAL x BMR.

triaclyglycerol (TAG) The major dietary fat, made of a glycerol backbone and three fatty acids (of which there are many different types), with the main division being between saturated and unsaturated types.

ENERGY

the 30-second digest

Our body uses energy to fuel cellular metabolism, especially the major organs like brain, heart, liver and gastrointestinal tract, and for physical activity. Carbohydrates and proteins each provide 17 kJ/g of metabolizable energy intake, with fats and alcohol providing 37 kJ/g and 29 kJ/g respectively. Our appetite mechanism usually allows us to match energy intake to energy expenditure so that we maintain a healthy body weight, but when we overeat, the excess energy intake is stored as fat. Overweight people should aim for an energy intake slightly less than their energy expenditure so that their energy deficit is met from their body fat, helping them to achieve a lower, healthy body weight. Our total energy expenditure (TEE) depends on the rate at which the body expends energy at rest (basal metabolic rate – BMR) and our physical activity level (PAL), and this is expressed by the relationship: TEE = PAL x BMR. BMR can be predicted from body weight, sex and age, and PAL varies with lifestyle from 1.35 in sedentary people to 2.5 for the very active. At an average PAL of 1.63, men and women of average height need 11 MJ and 9 MJ of food energy each day for a healthy body weight.

RELATED TOPICS

See also
DIGESTION & ABSORPTION
page 36

METABOLISM
page 38

OVERWEIGHT & OBESITY
page 86

3-SECOND BIOGRAPHIES

WILBUR OLIN ATWATER
1844–1907
American chemist who built the first whole body calorimeter to measure energy expenditure.

FRANCIS GANO BENEDICT
1870–1957
Chemist who worked with Atwater and invented a respirometer, to measure human oxygen consumption.

DALE SCHOELLER
1951–
The first to measure energy expenditure in humans using isotopically-labelled water.

30-SECOND TEXT
D Joe Millward

The amount of energy a food contains per gram is known as its energy density.

3-SECOND BITE
Macronutrients in food, beverages and alcohol fuel metabolism, organ function and physical activity, resulting in consumption of oxygen and production of heat and carbon dioxide (CO_2).

3-MINUTE SNACK
There is obvious variation between individuals in body shape, yet everyone conforms to the energy balance principle that food energy intake is balanced by energy expenditure plus any gain or loss of body energy stores, i.e. weight change. Both food energy intake and all components of energy expenditure are difficult to measure accurately and some commentators, especially authors of dieting plans, challenge the energy balance principle. However, rigorous measurements show that energy balance is always evident.

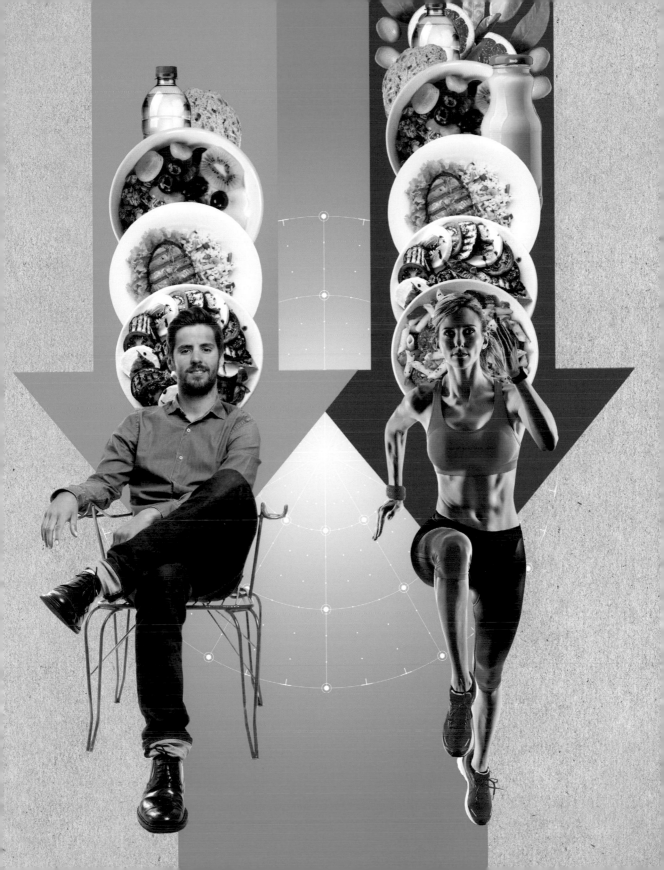

PROTEIN

the 30-second digest

3-SECOND BITE
The human genome codes the sequences of all 21 amino acids in 19,000–20,000 proteins, determining all aspects of the structure and function of the body.

3-MINUTE SNACK
We need dietary amino acids to make new proteins during growth and to make various other molecules, such as hormones and neuro-transmitters. Although all proteins are continuously degraded and replaced during protein turnover, the amino acids are mainly recycled, so turnover does not generate much dietary demand. Apart from the needs for new protein during childhood growth, pregnancy and lactation, our minimum dietary amino-acid needs are usually small, sufficient to make the various non-protein molecules.

Perhaps the ultimate building block, protein provides all the functional and structural components of the body: skin, bone, muscle, blood and all the organs. It consists of one or more long chains of amino acids linked by peptide bonds. Essential in the diet, protein provides the amino acids that are reassembled to build new body tissue during growth, used to maintain existing protein structures and to make smaller molecules like hormones and neurotransmitters. It can also serve as a fuel for the body – with the same energy density as carbohydrates (4 kal/17 kJ per gram). Protein is present in all foods – animal and plant – but rich sources include meats, dairy, fish, eggs, grains, legumes and nuts. The key is to eat a variety of these foods, to make sure that we absorb the right balance of the nine essential and the non-essential amino acids. This can be done with plant-based diets, as evident by the normal growth patterns of children in affluent vegan communities. The minimum dietary requirement of protein is for sufficient amino-acid nitrogen and indispensable amino acids to meet the demand for any growth, pregnancy or lactation and for body maintenance, balancing all nitrogen losses mainly through urea excretion. The minimum demand is usually small, and is easily met in most nutritionally complete diets.

RELATED TOPICS
See also
ENERGY
page 14

NUTS
page 62

VEGAN & VEGETARIANISM
page 66

3-SECOND BIOGRAPHIES
RUSSELL HENRY CHITTENDEN
1856–1943
Professor of physiological chemistry at Yale who revolutionized scientific thought on human protein requirements, showing that health and athletic performance required only modest intakes of protein.

WILLIAM CUMMING ROSE
1887–1985
American biochemist and nutritionist who discovered the amino acid threonine and determined the amount of each essential amino acid required to maintain nitrogen balance.

30-SECOND TEXT
D Joe Millward

More protein is required for rehabilitation after illness or after very strenuous exercise.

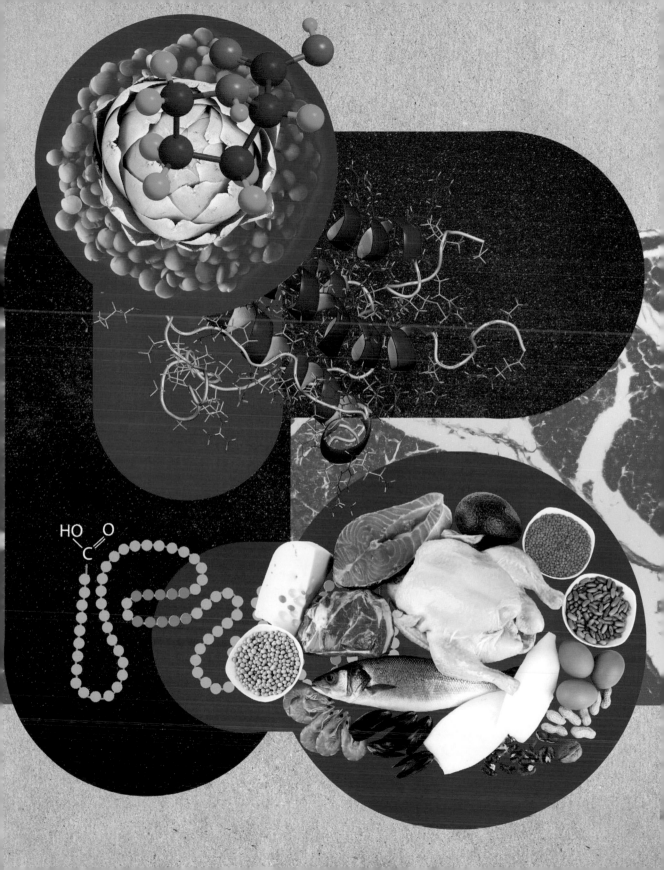

CARBOHYDRATES

the 30-second digest

Carbohydrates are one of the three main components of the diet (the macronutrients) and provide the major substrate for energy metabolism within the brain, kidney medulla and red blood cells. Carbohydrates are also important for muscle function in high-intensity exercise. Whilst dietary carbohydrates can range from molecules such as glucose and fructose (the simple sugars), through the disaccharides (sucrose, maltose, lactose) to the complex polymers of glucose found in starch, all dietary forms are digested within the intestine so that the simple sugars are the molecules that are absorbed into the body. Dietary recommendations for healthy people suggest carbohydrates should provide between 45 and 60% of dietary energy, depending on age, physical activity and body weight. High intakes of the simple sugars, sucrose or maltose, and even rapidly digested refined grains, are associated with risks to health, including tooth decay and unintentional overconsumption of energy (leading to weight gain). A healthy diet should have most carbohydrate in the complex form, particularly when contained in high-fibre wholegrain cereals and vegetables. The idea that carbohydrate is somehow toxic and that low-carbohydrate diets should be eaten by all is not backed up by research.

3-SECOND BITE
Carbohydrates are essential for health, but this does not mean that high-sugar foods are healthy.

3-MINUTE SNACK
It is frequently stated that carbohydrates are bad and 'low carb' diets are healthier than higher carbohydrate diets. Much of this arises from long-term prospective cohort studies which ignore the type of carbohydrate consumed. Clearly, high-sugars and refined-grain diets are not advisable, but diets high in fibre, wholegrain and low glycaemic index foods are not bad for you – in fact, the opposite is the case.

RELATED TOPICS
See also
ENERGY
page 14

FIBRE
page 20

SUGAR & SUGAR SUBSTITUTES
page 106

3-SECOND BIOGRAPHIES
CARL & GERTY CORI
1896–1984 & 1896–1957
The Czech–American couple's research into carbohydrate metabolism resulted in their sharing the Nobel Prize.

PROFESSOR RUSSELL KEAST
Lead researcher from a team in Australia which showed that there is a 'sixth taste' elicited by other carbohydrates independent of sweet taste. Those who are sensitive to the taste are thought to gravitate to carb-rich foods.

30-SECOND TEXT
Ian Macdonald

When consumed in the right foods, carbs are important contributors to health.

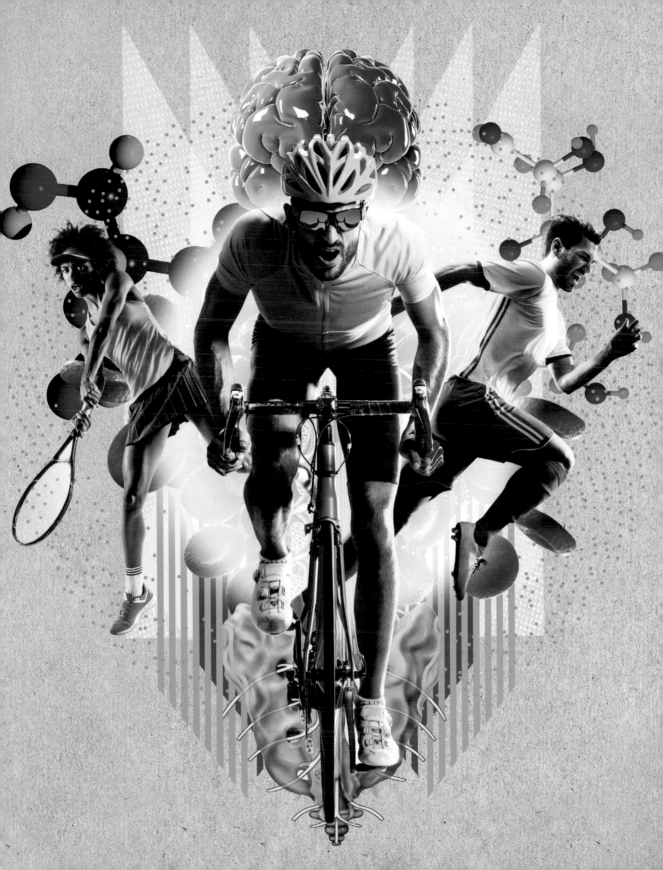

FIBRE

the 30-second digest

Dietary fibre is the indigestible component of foods and drinks which has a bulking effect in the large intestine and provides a substrate for the colonic bacteria. Originally, 'fibre' was limited to non-starch polysaccharides (such as cellulose) plus lignin from plants. In recent years the definition of fibre has widened to include all food components that are not digested and absorbed in the small intestine, including the non-digestible oligosaccharides (which are between the simple sugars and the starch polymers) and resistant starch. There is also an increasing use of novel, synthetic fibres in processed foods and drinks. Recent research suggests that a high intake of dietary fibre, particularly cereal fibre and whole grains, is associated with a reduced risk of cardiometabolic disease and colorectal cancer. Higher intakes of some fibre components are also associated with reductions in serum cholesterol and triacylglycerols as well as blood pressure. As a result, in recent years many countries have raised the recommended intake of dietary fibre to 30 grams (1 oz) or more for adults – almost twice the average present intake. The novel fibres, such as polydextrose, are of potential benefit, but evidence is needed to show that they have beneficial effects in the people consuming them.

RELATED TOPICS
See also
DIGESTION & ABSORPTION
page 36

GUT MICROBIOME
page 40

FRUIT & VEGETABLES
page 54

3-SECOND BIOGRAPHIES
HUGH CAREY TROWELL
1904–89
Identified dietary fibre as the vitally healthy substance in plant foods missing from industrialized Western diet.

DENIS PARSONS BURKITT
1911–93
Irish surgeon who compared diseases in African hospitals with Western diseases, concluding that many Western diseases were the result of diet and lifestyle.

30-SECOND TEXT
Ian Macdonald

Promotion of high-fibre diets should be an important part of health guidelines.

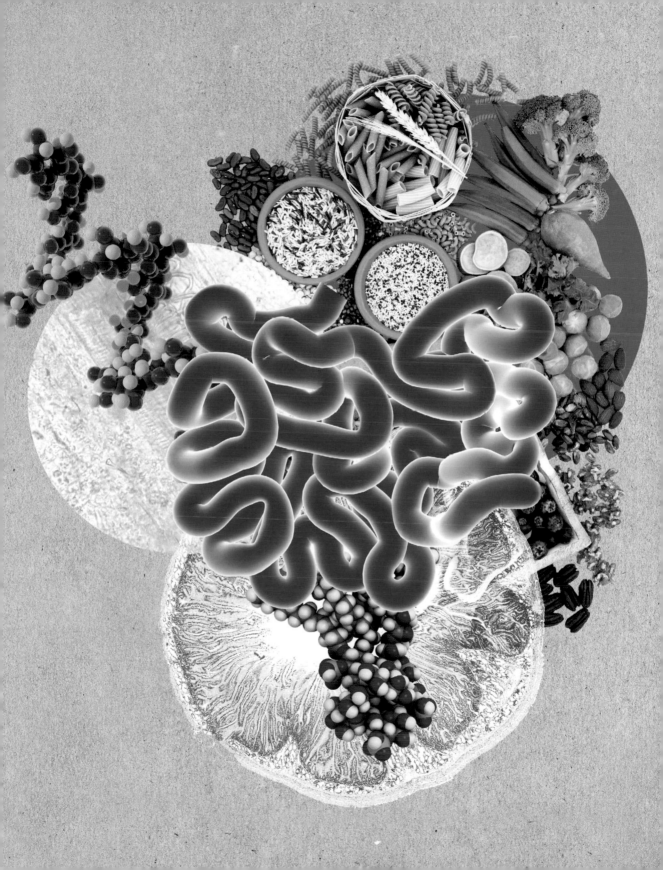

FATS

the 30-second digest

Fat is familiar to us as a substance we eat in food and store in our body. Both have the same chemical structure known as triaclyglycerol (TAG), which, when over-consumed in food, accumulates as body fat and increases body weight. The average 70-kg (155-lb) man has about 15 kg (33 lb) of body fat, which is equivalent to 140,000 calories or 40 days of stored energy, but only 0.3 kg (10 oz) of stored carbohydrate (900 calories). The physical and chemical properties of fats (TAG) in food are determined by differences in their component fatty acids (FAs), which differ in size and number of carbon double bonds. Saturated fats are mainly derived from animal sources and are solid at room temperature due to a lack of double bonds (such as butter), while monounsaturated fats have one, and polyunsaturated fats have two or more double bonds, which turn these fats into liquid oils. These oils can be extracted from plant seeds, including flax, olive and sunflower. The human body can make all but two FAs, namely linoleic acid and alpha-linolenic acid, so these fats must be acquired in our diet and are called 'essential fatty acids'. Fatty acids are used as building blocks for cell membranes in the body and to make hormone-like compounds (eicosanoids) that have metabolic effects essential for life.

3-MINUTE SNACK
Dietary fats are less filling and provide more than twice the energy per gram than carbohydrates and proteins, properties that increase its potential to increase body weight. While most saturated fats come from animal products, one notable exception is coconut oil, which is a highly saturated, hard vegetable fat.

RELATED TOPICS
See also
METABOLISM
page 38

DIETARY FATS &
HEART DISEASE
page 98

3-SECOND BIOGRAPHIES
WILLIAM PROUT
1785–1850
English physician and chemist who was one of the first to recognize the importance of fat as a nutrient in our diet.

GEORGE BURR
1896–1990
American professor who, along with his wife, Mildred, discovered the first dietary FA that was essential for life, linoleic acid.

KONRAD BLOCK
1912–2000
Discovered, with Feodor Lynen, the mechanism and regulation of cholesterol and FA metabolism.

30-SECOND TEXT
Bruce A Griffin

Coconut oil is high in saturated fat (85%), while butter is 50% and olive oil is 10%.

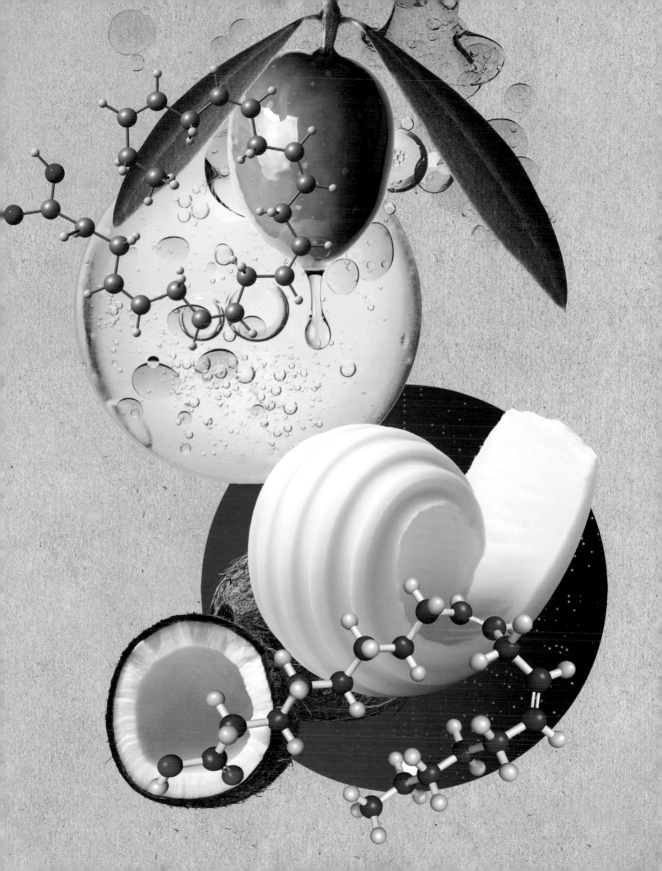

MINERALS

the 30-second digest

Minerals are inorganic substances that are not made by living things. Found in both soil and rocks, they are absorbed by plants that are then eaten. Minerals are largely classified as 'major' minerals or 'trace' minerals. Major minerals are those that the body requires in amounts of at least 100 mg per day, and include sodium, potassium, calcium, magnesium, sulphur, phosphorus and chloride. Trace minerals are needed in amounts of less than 100 mg per day, and some, such as iron, fluoride, zinc and manganese, have established recommended daily allowances (RDAs) or Adequate Intake (AI) limits to ensure adequacy. A third classification, known as 'ultra-trace' minerals, require less than 1 mg per day, and include chromium, copper, iodine, molybdenum and selenium. Minerals play a role in maintaining a healthy immune system, bone and teeth health, muscle contraction, fluid balance and overall growth. A healthy diet of fruits, vegetables, whole grains and lean meats is one way to ensure adequate intake of minerals; supplementation is another way. While deficiencies may present detrimental health conditions, it is important to be aware of intake amounts when supplementing, to avoid toxicity symptoms such as nausea and vomiting, which may occur with overconsumption.

3-SECOND BITE
Common food sources for minerals are beans, peas, dairy, eggs, cereals, fruit, meat, poultry, vegetables, whole grains and seafood.

3-MINUTE SNACK
Iron deficiency anaemia is the most common mineral disorder in the world. It is estimated that over 30% of the world's population are considered anaemic, including 40% of pre-school children in developing countries. Major health consequences include impaired physical and cognitive development, increased risk of morbidity in children and reduced productivity in adults. Iron-rich foods, fortification and supplementation help to relieve symptoms.

RELATED TOPICS
See also
FRUIT & VEGETABLES
page 54

SALT & BLOOD PRESSURE
page 104

3-SECOND BIOGRAPHY
HUMPHRY DAVY
1778–1829
Cornish chemist and inventor who was the first to successfully isolate calcium in 1808, by electrolysing lime in mercury oxide.

30-SECOND TEXT
Jill Snyder

Minerals can compete with each another in the absorption process, which takes place in the small intestine.

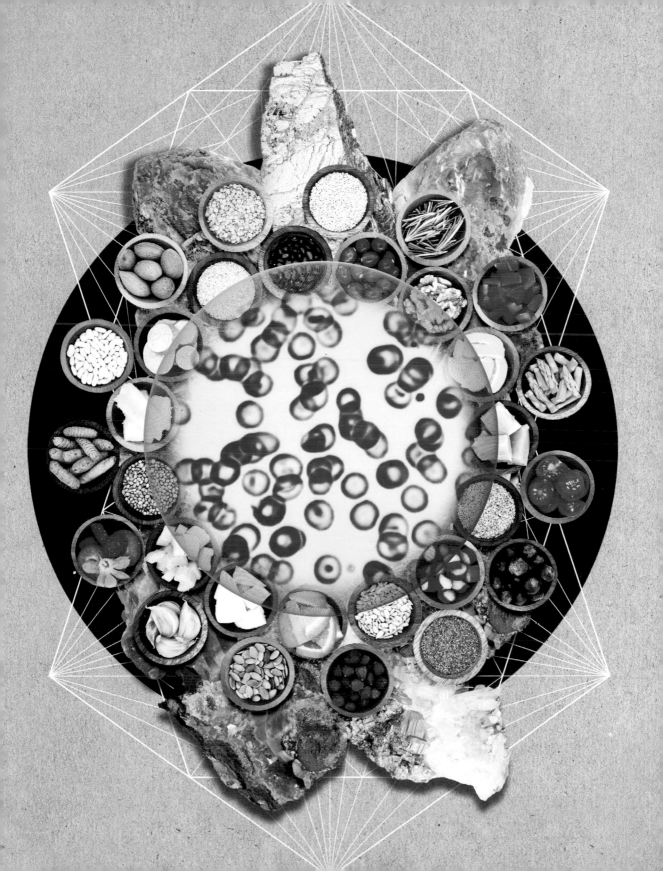

FAT-SOLUBLE VITAMINS

the 30-second digest

Vitamins A, D, E and K comprise a small group of fat-soluble vitamins of disparate chemical composition which are essential for good health. Various processes are dependent on an adequate availability of these vitamins, including vision (vitamin A), growth and tissue differentiation (vitamins A and D), bone and muscle function (vitamin D), immune function (vitamin A), protection against free radicals (vitamin E) and blood clotting (vitamin K). Although fat-soluble vitamins can be stored in the body for use in times of dietary scarcity, deficiencies do occur, with profound consequences. In some regions of the world, young children are at risk of becoming blind because of inadequate vitamin A. Vitamin D deficiency, which is common worldwide, may cause bowed legs and pelvic deformities of rickets in children and muscle weakness and bone pain of osteomalacia in adults. Foods of animal origin tend to be good sources of fat-soluble vitamins, but red, yellow and orange vegetables are an excellent source of carotenoids (a form of vitamin A), and vitamins E and K are found in nuts and seeds. Vitamin D is unusual as humans can synthesize it through sunlight on skin, which is important because only a few foods are rich in vitamin D.

3-SECOND BITE
Fat-soluble vitamins are essential to life, but too little or too much in our diet may have profound adverse health effects.

3-MINUTE SNACK
High-dose supplements of some fat-soluble vitamins can have severe adverse effects. High-dose supplements of vitamin D can actually increase fracture risk and may cause damage to the heart and kidneys. Vitamin A is toxic at high doses, causing serious birth defects and possibly fractures. In smokers, too much beta-carotene (a form of vitamin A) may even increase the risk of death from lung cancer.

RELATED TOPICS
See also
WATER-SOLUBLE VITAMINS
page 28

MALNUTRITION
page 88

VITAMIN D & CALCIUM
page 126

3-SECOND BIOGRAPHIES
FREDERICK GOWLAND HOPKINS
1861–1947
British biochemist who demonstrated that components in milk were essential for normal growth in rats, which paved the way to characterizing individual vitamins.

HENRIK DAM
1895–1976
Danish scientist who discovered a dietary factor that promoted blood clotting. This factor was vitamin K.

30-SECOND TEXT
Hilary Powers

Fat-soluble vitamins are usually absorbed in fat globules that travel through the lymphatic system.

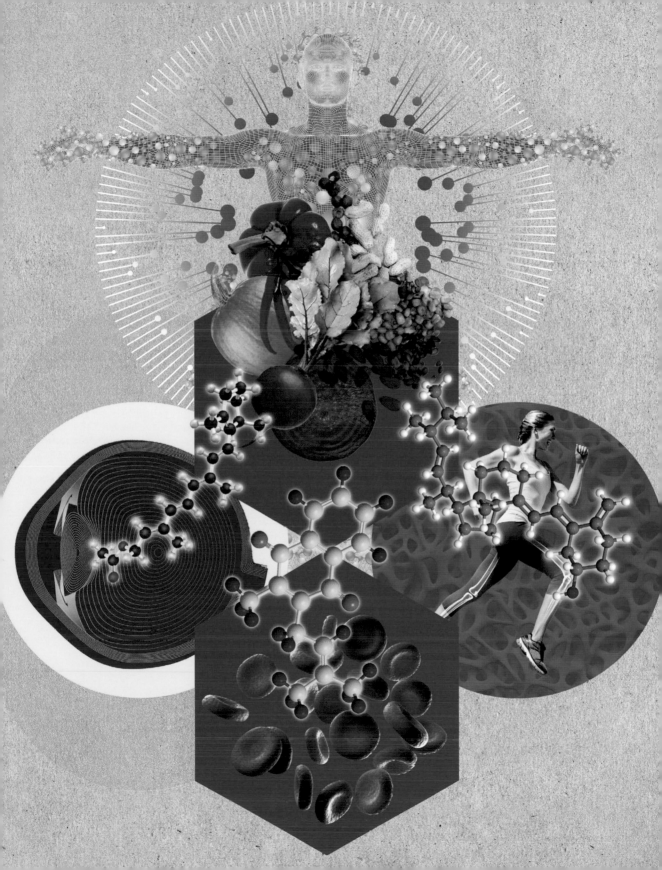

WATER-SOLUBLE VITAMINS

the 30-second digest

3-SECOND BITE

Water-soluble vitamins comprise a disparate group of compounds needed in small amounts in the human diet, to carry out a wide range of essential functions in the body.

3-MINUTE SNACK

Claims that high-dose supplements of water-soluble vitamins confer special health benefits, or help us to live longer, are generally not well-founded. Although people with poor diets or higher requirements may need vitamin supplements to prevent symptoms of deficiency, supplement use is most common amongst healthy people consuming a varied and nutritious diet. Indeed, very high-dose vitamin supplement use may have adverse health effects, including a possible increase in cancer risk.

Water-soluble vitamins perform a wide range of important functions, including the extraction of energy from food, cell signalling, synthesis of DNA and conduction of nerve impulses. Water-soluble vitamins comprise nine compounds – vitamins B_1, B_2, B_6, B_{12}, C, niacin, folate, biotin and pantothenic acid – distinguished by their chemistry and function. They are required regularly in small amounts in the human diet as they are not stored in the body; excess intake is removed by the kidneys. Symptoms of deficiency may occur if a diet lacks any one of these vitamins. For example, a diet lacking in vitamin C can lead to the development of scurvy, characterized by impaired wound healing, joint pain, tiredness and shortness of breath; a diet lacking in vitamin B12 may lead to anaemia and degeneration of the spinal cord. It has proved difficult to know exactly how much of each vitamin is required daily to stay healthy. Early experiments (that would be considered unethical today), systematically deprived human volunteers of vitamin C to determine how much of this vitamin reversed symptoms of scurvy. Such studies formed the basis of dietary reference values for water-soluble vitamins. A varied diet that includes fruit and vegetables, cereals, meat, fish and dairy products is likely to satisfy a person's requirements.

RELATED TOPICS

See also
FAT-SOLUBLE VITAMINS
page 26

METABOLISM
page 38

MALNUTRITION
page 88

3-SECOND BIOGRAPHY

LUCY WILLS
1888–1964
English medical scientist who demonstrated that a factor in yeast extract cured pernicious anaemia of pregnancy. This heralded the discovery of the vitamin folate.

30-SECOND TEXT

Hilary Powers

A regular supply of each water-soluble vitamin is needed to avoid developing deficiency disease.

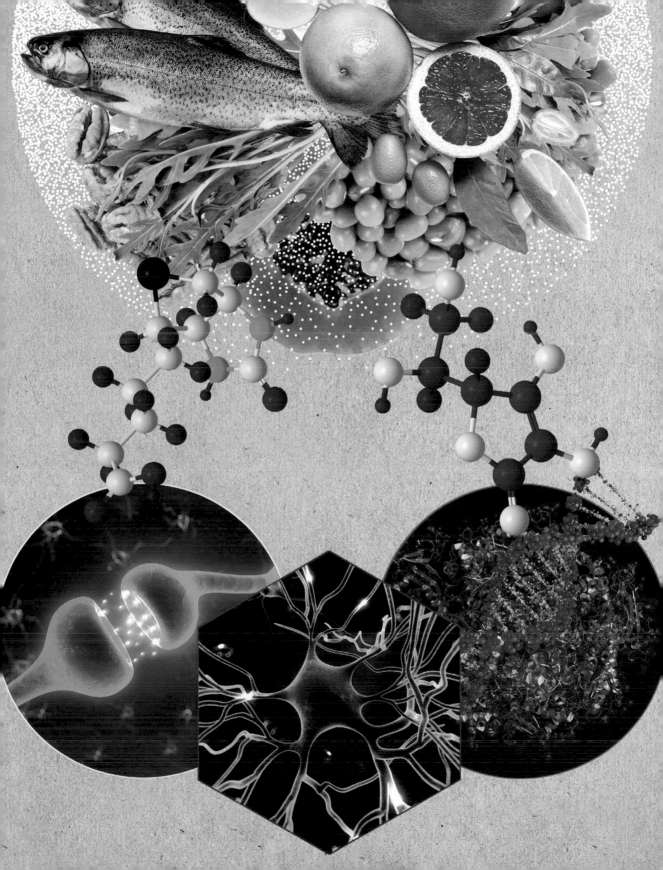

20 June 1861
Born in Eastbourne, UK

1878
Graduates from school in Enfield

1883
Works at the Home Office as an assistant to Sir Thomas Stevenson.

1894
Graduates in Medicine from Guy's Hospital, London, and achieves his doctoral degree

1898
Marries Jessie Anne Stevens, with whom he goes on to have two daughters

1907
With Sir Walter Morley, discovers the role of lactic acid in muscle contractions

1912
Coins the word 'vitamin' after conducting a series of animal feeding experiments

1914
Becomes Chair of Biochemistry at Cambridge University, the first person in the country to hold that position

1929
Awarded the Nobel Prize in Physiology for Medicine with Christiaan Eijkman

16 May 1947
Dies in Cambridge and is buried at the Parish of the Ascension Burial Ground

SIR FREDERICK GOWLAND HOPKINS

Fans of vitamins can thank Sir Frederick Hopkins for their early discovery. His vital research over the years shone a light on the 'accessory food factors', later named vitamins, which had an enormous impact on growth and function in living things, despite being present in tiny amounts in the diet.

Sir Frederick was born in Eastbourne in 1861 where he was raised by his mother and uncle; his bookseller father having died when Sir Frederick was a baby. Ten years later, the family moved to Enfield in North London, where he excelled in science, particularly chemistry.

The first big break came in 1883, when Sir Frederick was offered a post at the Home Office to work on poisons alongside Sir Thomas Stevenson. This led him to complete a BSc in chemistry followed by a medical degree at Guy's Hospital, London. After graduating, he continued at Guy's to teach physiology and toxicology, during which time he developed research into what would become the new discipline of biochemistry. Early experiments revealed the workings of muscle before Sir Frederick's attention switched to nutrition, another under-developed topic.

A move to Cambridge University in 1898 began a period of intense research, culminating in the work that made his name. Sir Frederick's first success was to isolate the amino acid, tryptophan, from protein and prove that certain amino acids could not be manufactured by the body. This led to the concept of 'essential' amino acids. Further research on laboratory animals revealed that the prevalent view of a balanced diet – one that contained sufficient proteins, fats, carbohydrates, minerals and water – was lacking something vital. His papers in 1906 and 1912 are acknowledged as the first to develop the theory on the importance of vitamins.

Subsequently, after building on research by Christiaan Eijkman, Sir Frederick discovered that thiamin in unprocessed rice could reverse the deficiency disease beriberi. For this work, he and Eijkman were awarded the 1929 Nobel Prize. Further research delved into the biochemistry of cells and enzymes, adding many useful findings to human knowledge. Honours rapidly followed: the Royal Medal of the Royal Society of London in 1918; a knighthood in 1925; and the Order of Merit in 1935. Until his death, Sir Frederick continued to influence his peers and oversaw the flourishing of the two disciplines that he had nurtured during his lifetime.

Carrie Ruxton

NUTRIENTS: CONSUMPTION & METABOLISM

amines Derivatives of ammonia; released by the breakdown of amino acids. Many neurotransmitters are amines, including dopamine, serotonin and histamine. Can be found in cheese, wine and chocolate, for example.

APOE gene Provides instructions for making a protein called apolipoprotein E. APOE genotyping is sometimes used to help in the diagnosis of late-onset Alzheimer disease.

dextrin Common food additive, used as a thickening and preservative agent. Produced by heating any starch in the presence of either water or a dilute hydrochloric acid. Not all forms are digestible; indigestible dextrin is sometimes used in fibre supplements.

enzymes Protein molecules in cells which work as catalysts, speeding up chemical reactions in the body. Essential to life.

epidemiology The study of how often diseases occur in different populations and why.

fatty acids The building blocks of fat in the body and in food. During digestion, the body breaks down fats into fatty acids, which can then be absorbed into the blood. Essential fatty acids (EFAs) must be ingested because the body requires them for good health but cannot synthesize them. Those not essential are non-essential fatty acids.

Human Genome Project International research collaboration, from 1990 to 2003, to map and understand the genes of human beings.

lipids Another word for 'fats'. Contain carbon, hydrogen and oxygen. Along with carbohydrates and proteins, lipids are the main constituents of cells and are easily stored in the body and used as a source of fuel.

maltose Also known as malt sugar. Made out of two glucose molecules bound together, it's created in seeds and other parts of plants. Cereals, certain fruits and sweet potatoes contain high amounts.

metabolites Products of metabolism; substances essential to the metabolism of a particular organism or to a particular metabolic process.

microbiome Gut microbiome is a vast ecosystem of organisms such as bacteria, yeasts, fungi, viruses and protozoans that live in our digestive pipes. Many of these organisms are vital – breaking down food and toxins, making vitamins and training our immune systems. Currently subject to significant research.

nucleic acids Essential to all known forms of life, nucleic acids are the main information-carrying molecules of a cell and determine the inherited characteristics of every living thing. The two main classes deoxyribonucleic acid (DNA) and ribonucleic acid (RNA).

nutrigenetics The science of how nutritional components in our diet interact with variations in our genes.

obesity Significantly overweight, with excess body fat; commonly measured using body mass index (BMI). Generally caused when more calories are consumed than burned. The excess energy is stored by the body as fat. Can lead to diabetes, heart disease, cancer, stroke and depression.

polymorphisms Discontinuous genetic variation of a gene that may result in different characteristics or disease risk among the members of a single species.

polyphenols Abundant substances found in fruits, vegetables and nuts; evidence for their role in the prevention of degenerative diseases such as cancer and cardiovascular diseases is emerging.

prebiotic Substrate that beneficially affects the host by targeting indigenous gut bacteria thought to be positive. Currently, main prebiotic targets are **bifidobacteria** and **lactobacilli**.

DIGESTION & ABSORPTION

the 30-second digest

The oral cavity, or mouth, is where food is initially broken up. Salivary enzymes, such as amylases and microbiota, aid this process by breaking down some starches into maltose and dextrin, and thereby starting the digestion process. In the stomach, a very low pH further degrades foods, and microbial populations are maintained at relatively low levels. Gastric juice in the stomach starts protein digestion. The small intestine is a very narrow tube with a large surface area and is the major site of absorption in humans – in fact, 95% of absorption of nutrients occurs here. Pancreatic enzymes and bile aid the digestive process and microbial numbers begin to rise. Finally, the transit time of the large intestine is very slow, with around 200 g of dietary contents entering per day in an adult. The dietary contents are a mixture of undigested carbohydrates, proteins, vitamins and lipids. These help to fortify an intensively colonized microbiota, which contributes to digestion by metabolizing these substrates into organic acids, gases and nitrogenous compounds like ammonia, amines and phenols. Each of these may exert varying influences upon health.

RELATED TOPICS

See also
METABOLISM
page 38

GUT MICROBIOME
page 40

3-SECOND BITE
The gastrointestinal tract (GIT) is comprised of anatomically distinct areas. The digestive system starts in the oral cavity, progressing through the oesophagus to the stomach and small and large intestines.

3-MINUTE SNACK
Bacteria in the human gastrointestinal tract, also called 'gut flora' or 'microbiome', help with digestion. The total number of microorganisms present is about 1014, with the overall microbiome gene pool being approximately 100 times greater than the human genome – by far the majority being colonic.

3-SECOND BIOGRAPHIES
WILLIAM BEAUMONT
1785–1853
US Army surgeon who became known as the 'Father of Gastric Physiology', constructing over 200 experiments to provide new information about gastric physiology and the digestive process in human beings.

CLAUDE BERNARD
1813–78
French physiologist who verified that the small intestine was the major site of digestion and that pancreatic secretions were important digestive agents.

30-SECOND TEXT
Katherine Stephens
& Glenn Gibson

Starting in the mouth, our food goes through a lengthy process to be digested and absorbed.

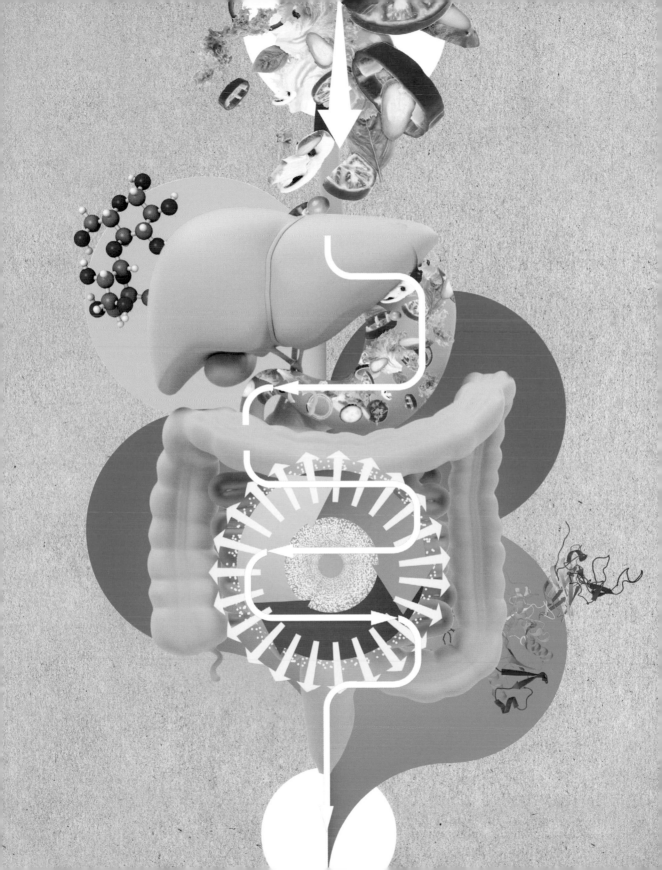

METABOLISM

the 30-second digest

Metabolism can be defined as the chemical processes by which organisms convert food into energy to maintain life, growth and to reproduce. These processes occur inside and outside of cells in the body and can be 'destructive' (catabolic) processes, which release energy by breaking down large molecules into their constituent parts (dietary fats, carbohydrates and protein) to provide the fuel for 'constructive' (anabolic) processes, which involve building large complex molecules for structural and functional roles in living organisms (proteins, fats and nucleic acids). These processes occur in a series of energy-dependent steps, whereby one molecule such as glucose is broken down into smaller molecules to release energy, or, conversely, molecules are built-up to make larger molecules. These series of transformative steps are called 'metabolic pathways' and are regulated by enzymes (proteins that act as chemical catalysts) that promote reactions to convert substrates into products, which would not happen spontaneously. The activity of enzymes can be controlled in many different ways to regulate metabolism (rate or flux of molecule transformations through the pathway). The rate of metabolism can be estimated by measuring the rate at which energy is used by an organism.

RELATED TOPICS
See also
ENERGY
page 14

CARBOHYDRATES
page 18

FAT
page 22

3-SECOND BIOGRAPHIES
HANS KREBS
1900–81
Professor of Biochemistry at Oxford who shared a Nobel Prize for his part in the discovery of a key metabolic pathway that explains how energy is derived from carbohydrate, fats and proteins.

KONRAD BLOCH
1912–2000
Professor of Biochemistry at Harvard who won a Nobel Prize for his part in the discovery of the mechanism and regulation of cholesterol and fatty acid biosynthesis.

30-SECOND TEXT
Bruce A Griffin

The 'resting metabolic rate' measures the energy required to maintain the body.

3-SECOND BITE
A popular misconception is that humans become obese because they have slow metabolism, but obese humans have a higher metabolic rate than non-obese humans.

3-MINUTE SNACK
Eating less food energy and physical activity have marked and immediate effects on metabolism, which, if sustained, will result in reduced body weight over time. However, there is no evidence that specific foods or nutrients can accelerate or boost metabolism to promote weight loss. On the contrary, there is evidence for the existence of differences in metabolism between groups of individuals, known as 'metabotypes', to which dietary recommendations can be specifically tailored to improve benefits to health.

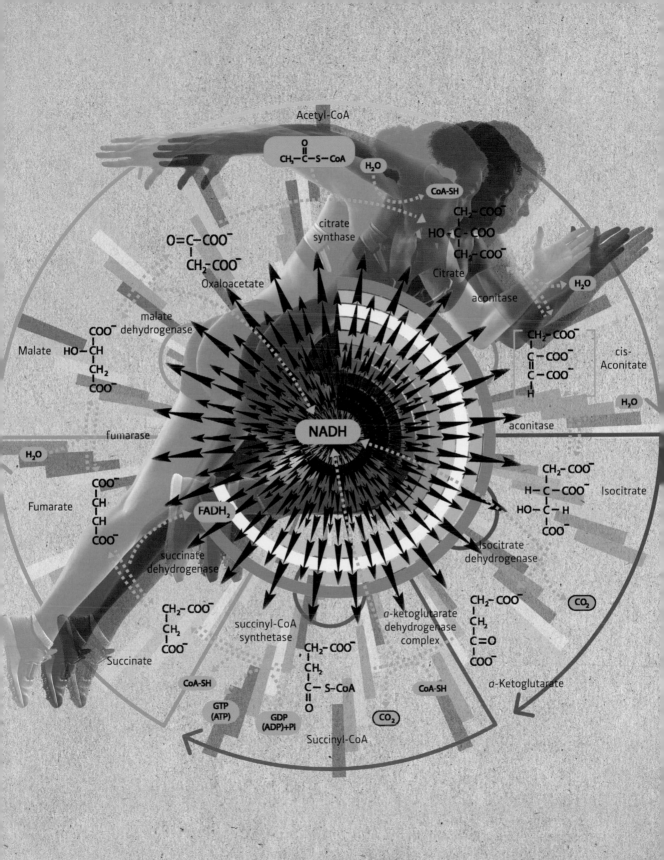

GUT MICROBIOME

the 30-second digest

The gut microbiome is a vast ecosystem of organisms such as bacteria, yeasts, fungi and viruses that live in our digestive pipes. Many of these organisms are vital – breaking down food and toxins, making vitamins and training our immune systems. Gut transit time and pH maintain gut microbiota populations in the stomach and small intestine at lower levels than in the large intestine, where the vast majority of microbiota reside. Metabolic capacity of the microbiota is vast, with many different end products being formed, including short-chain fatty acids (SCFA). These are thought to exert energy generation, satiety and colonocyte regulation. Fermentable carbohydrates like starch and fibres are the main substrates for SCFA generation. On the contrary, protein and lipids can be metabolized by the microbiota, but these produce toxic compounds such as ammonia and certain amines. Through the formation of metabolites, microbiota end products can onset intolerance symptoms. The indigenous microbiome can influence the immune response both positively and negatively. More positive components of gut microbiota can be fortified: a prebiotic (such as *bifidobacteria* and *lactobacilli*) is a substrate that beneficially affects the host by targeting indigenous components thought to be positive.

3-SECOND BITE
Diet provides the main growth substrates for gut microbiota, some of which are positive for health; others are pathogenic, and the remainder are neutral.

3-MINUTE SNACK
The human intestinal tract is an intensively colonized area containing bacteria that are health-positive and benign, as well as pathogenic (causing disease). In fact, there are far more bacterial cells in the human body than there are mammalian ones. We are given our gut bugs during birth – the first, and one of the most important, presents of our life. They then go on to play a major role in digestion and health.

RELATED TOPICS
See also
PROTEIN
page 16

DIGESTION & ABSORPTION
page 36

PROBIOTICS & PREBIOTICS
page 128

3-SECOND BIOGRAPHY
JOHN CRYAN
Neuroscientist at the University College of Cork, Ireland, who has investigated how the gut microbiome affects the mammalian brain – with far-reaching public health implications.

30-SECOND TEXT
Glenn Gibson

In terms of effect on health, our gut bugs can be broadly categorized into the good, the bad and the indifferent.

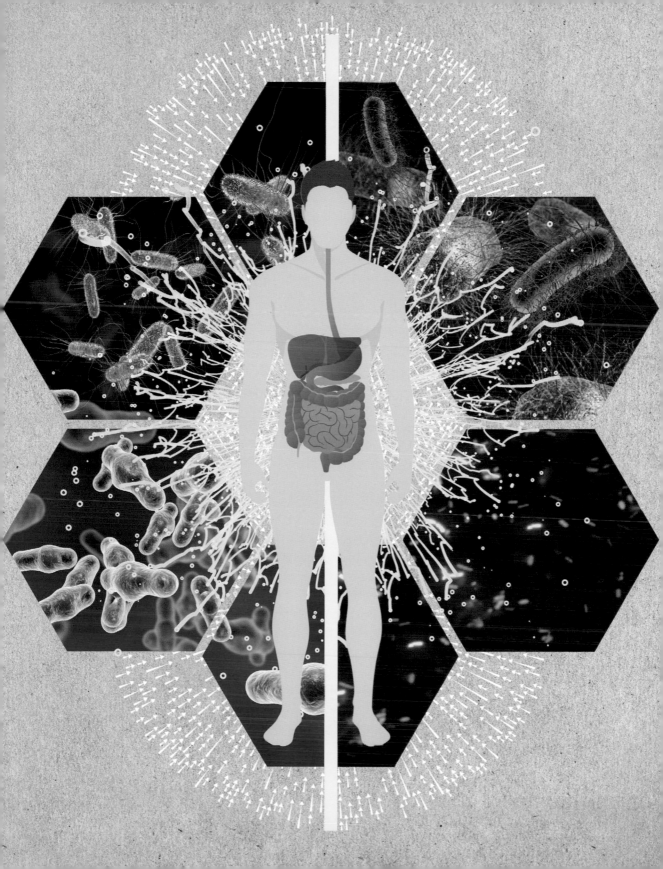

NUTRIENT-GENE INTERACTIONS

the 30-second digest

Nutrigenetics is the science of

how nutritional components in our diet interact with variations in our genes. People respond in different ways to eating certain kinds of foods, and this is because we all possess versions and combinations of genes. Sometimes copies of genes don't function or are damaged, which can lead to obesity, metabolic diseases, or even cancer. Versions of genes (or polymorphisms) involved with regulating our body weight, for example, can lead to some people gaining weight or becoming obese. Research has shown that individuals with a lower body mass index tend to eat more legumes, fruit and fish; and it is not so much how many calories a person consumes, but rather where those calories are coming from. Vitamins and minerals also play a key role in regulating our body's development and growth. Having enough B vitamins and folic acid within the diet can determine aspects of our overall health, as well as affect our risks of developing metabolic diseases. Consumption of certain foods can, however, decrease our risk of developing some diseases and improve our long-term health. Consuming polyphenols (found in fruits, vegetables and nuts) alters the expression of genes related to blood pressure, improving cardiovascular function, for instance.

3-SECOND BITE
Nutrient-gene interactions have a significant impact upon a person's likelihood of developing diseases such as cancer and cardiovascular disease in later life.

3-MINUTE SNACK
Nutrigenomics aims to understand how nutrients 'signal' and interact with genetic variation. Differences in genes, known as 'polymorphisms', can have significant impacts on a person's health. These 'genotypes' give rise to a person's 'phenotype', and dictate how nutrients are metabolized and excreted on a molecular level. Some people possess versions of genes that allow their cells to metabolize very efficiently; in others these genes might not function at all.

RELATED TOPICS
See also
METABOLISM
page 38

OVERWEIGHT & OBESITY
page 86

DIETARY FATS &
HEART DISEASE
page 98

3-SECOND BIOGRAPHY
JOSÉ M ORDOVÁS
1956–
A leading professor in the field of nutrient-gene interactions who has made an outstanding contribution to our understanding of the links between genetic variation and dietary response.

30-SECOND TEXT
Luke Bell

Understanding how our genes interact with nutrients could prevent some terminal diseases.

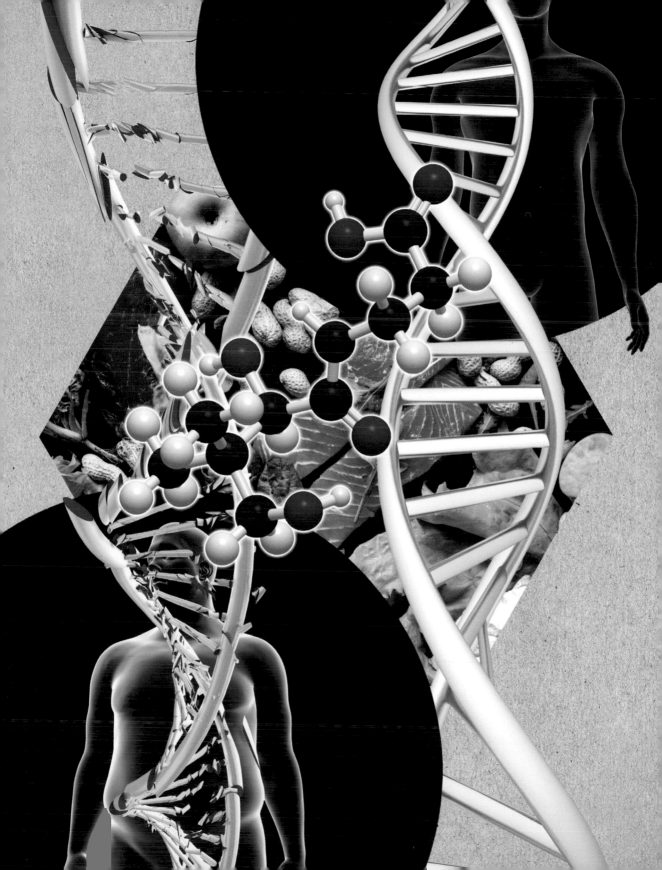

21 October 1906
Born in Wallington, UK

1928
Receives Bachelor of Science in Chemistry from Imperial College, London

1931
Receives Doctorate from University of London, having introduced new methodology for measuring the carbohydrate in apples

1933
Enrols for a Dietetics diploma course at King's College, London. Historic meeting with Robert McCance, her lifelong scientific partner, at King's College Hospital.

1938
Widdowson and McCance move to the Department of Experimental Medicine, Cambridge

1940
First edition of *The Chemical Composition of Foods* published

1946
An Experimental Study of Rationing is published, although the results had been made available to the British Government during WWII

1976
Elected as a Fellow of the Royal Society

1977–80
Elected President of the Nutrition Society

1979
Made a Commander of the British Empire (CBE)

1993
Made a Companion of Honour (CH), an honour restricted to only 65 Britons at any one time. Publication of biography, *McCance and Widdowson: a Scientific Partnership of 60 years* (Ed: Margaret Ashwell).

14 June 2000
Dies in Cambridge, UK

ELSIE WIDDOWSON

Although best known for her pioneering work on the first British food tables with her scientific partner for more than 60 years, Robert McCance, Elsie Widdowson's influence on nutrition went much further than the chemical composition of foods. She made significant scientific discoveries in the diverse worlds of mineral metabolism, body composition, the physiology of the newborn and in normal and retarded growth, to name just a few.

In the citation for her Honorary Doctorate, she was introduced as the woman who won World War II on account of her research for the British food rations. 'You can, if you have to, live on a very simple diet', she said. She worked out that bread, cabbage and potatoes contained all the nutrients for healthy survival in the event that Britain could not import food. For three months in 1939–40, Widdowson, McCance and a number of their companions ate nothing else. To demonstrate their fitness following this bleak regime, Elsie, McCance and two others completed a rigorous course of cycling and mountain climbing in the English Lake District. Just like the secret codebreakers of wartime Britain, Elsie was driven by Britain's desperate necessity to survive in wartime.

Self-experimentation featured highly in Elsie's research. Widdowson and McCance even came close to death once when they injected themselves with solutions to judge the absorption and excretion of minerals in the body. The photo of Elsie's arm jammed full of syringes never fails to wow today's students.

Elsie considered the most important unanswered question in nutrition to be the influence of genetics on the way that the body treats the nutrients delivered to it. She based her belief on her research of the individual diets of children in the 1930s and 40s, which had shown their vast range of energy and nutrient requirements: 'Similar individuals may differ enormously and unpredictably in their food habits.' These observations have paved the way to the modern study of nutrigenetics, now defined as the science of the effect of genetic variation on dietary response.

Promoting the acceptance and encouragement of women in science was Elsie's passion. On her death, the Imperial College Elsie Widdowson Fellowship Award was set up to allow academic staff to concentrate fully on their research work upon returning from maternity, adoption, surrogacy and/or shared parental leave.

Elsie always retained her humility, her intuition and her sense of excitement for discovery and debate. Her greatest satisfaction was discovering how something she had said, written or done had helped someone else in their career.

Margaret Ashwell

PERSONALIZED VERSUS PUBLIC HEALTH ADVICE

the 30-second digest

3-SECOND BITE
Personalized nutrition, tailored to an individual's diet intake, physical characteristics and genetic makeup has the potential to revolutionize the delivery of diet advice.

3-MINUTE SNACK
A key challenge in improving public health is motivating people to change their dietary behaviour. It is therefore vital that nutrition advice is personally relevant and easy to follow. In the future, researchers aim to harness technological advances, by combining complex personal data with smartphone applications and wearable technology, to provide effective personalized nutrition on a population-level.

Poor diet choices and lack of physical activity are some of the key causes of obesity, heart disease, diabetes and some cancers. Over the years, public health strategies have attempted to improve diet through campaigns, which are typically delivered on a population basis, using a 'one size fits all' approach. Guidelines may differ according to gender, age, weight or specific conditions such as pregnancy, and are unlikely to suit everybody. In contrast, personalized nutrition seeks to tailor dietary information according to individuals' characteristics, including diet intake and physical health. The completion of the Human Genome Project in 2003 made it possible to tailor advice based on genetic makeup. For example, research has shown that people with specific variants of the APOE gene respond better to a diet low in saturated fat. Motivating individuals to change their dietary behaviour is arguably one of the greatest challenges in nutrition interventions, and evidence suggests that an individualized approach – through a registered nutritionist/ dietitian – helps people to follow a healthy diet more than 'one size fits all' public health guidance. However, public health guidance remains a vital means of raising awareness of important health issues in the population.

RELATED TOPICS
See also
DIETARY ASSESSMENT
page 48

CHANGING EATING HABITS
page 92

3-SECOND BIOGRAPHY
JAMES WATSON
1928–
American molecular biologist and geneticist who co-discovered the structure of DNA in 1953 alongside Francis Crick and Rosalind Franklin, and helped establish the US arm of the Human Genome Project.

30-SECOND TEXT
Rosalind Fallaize

Personalized diet plans anchored in genetics could be the future for fighting health problems associated with poor nutrition.

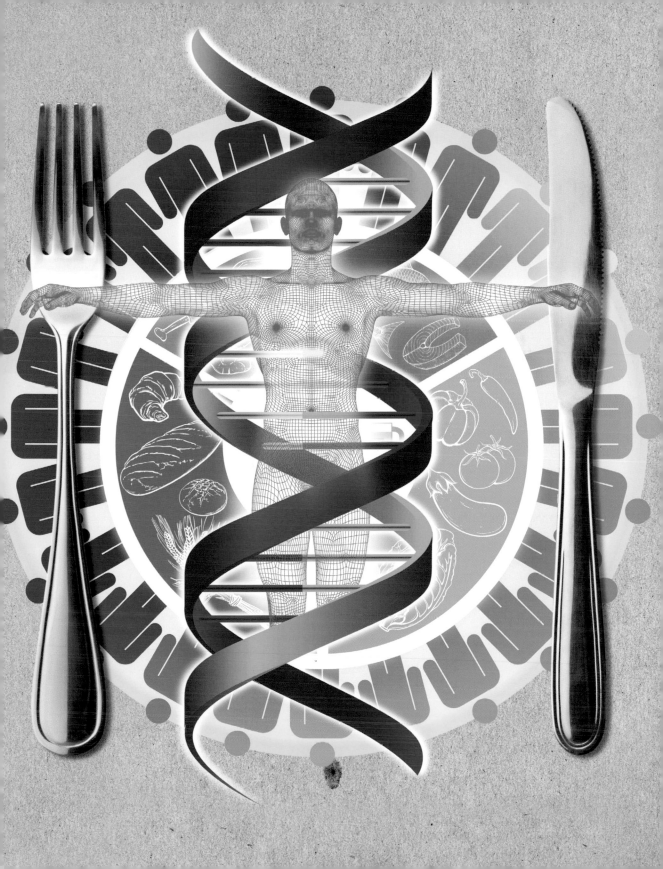

DIETARY ASSESSMENT

the 30-second digest

Scientists, healthcare professionals and, increasingly, members of the public are seeking new and innovative ways of assessing dietary intake. Accurate dietary assessment is vital, and forms an integral part of studies that focus on exploring the relationship between diet and health. Traditional methods of assessment include: food frequency questionnaires and diet recalls, whereby individuals are required to remember the foods they have eaten over the past 24 hours to one year; and food diaries, whereby individuals are asked to record what they eat in 'real time'. These traditional methods are often burdensome on both the individual and the researcher. Furthermore, individuals may under-report their food intake or change their dietary behaviour, because they are aware of being assessed. Several web-based tools have been developed to improve the accuracy of traditional assessment methods. In parallel, scientists are looking towards the use of biological markers in hair, urine, blood and faeces to assess dietary exposure. Commercial smartphone applications can help consumers to track their own dietary intake; however, further research is needed to assess the accuracy of these applications and their effectiveness for weight management.

3-SECOND BITE
Dietary assessment forms a vital part of nutritional science, and researchers are constantly exploring new and innovative ways of assessing energy and nutrient intake.

3-MINUTE SNACK
Technological advances have enabled the development of mobile dietary assessment instruments, which are easily incorporated into the user's lifestyle. Additionally, biological markers are being developed to assess nutritional status and recent dietary intake. While biological markers are expensive and do not reflect multiple dimensions of dietary intake, they have the capacity to validate and improve the accuracy of self-reported dietary assessment tools.

RELATED TOPICS
See also
PROFILE: ELSIE WIDDOWSON
page 44

PERSONALIZED VERSUS PUBLIC HEALTH ADVICE
page 46

CHANGING EATING HABITS
page 92

3-SECOND BIOGRAPHY
ELSIE WIDDOWSON
1906–2000
British dietitian who studied nutritional deficiencies and helped to revolutionize the way in which dietary intake could be explored relative to disease risk.

30-SECOND TEXT
Rosalind Fallaize & Oonagh Markey

Diet records provide insight into food habits and are used by dietitians/nutritionists to help individuals improve dietary intake.

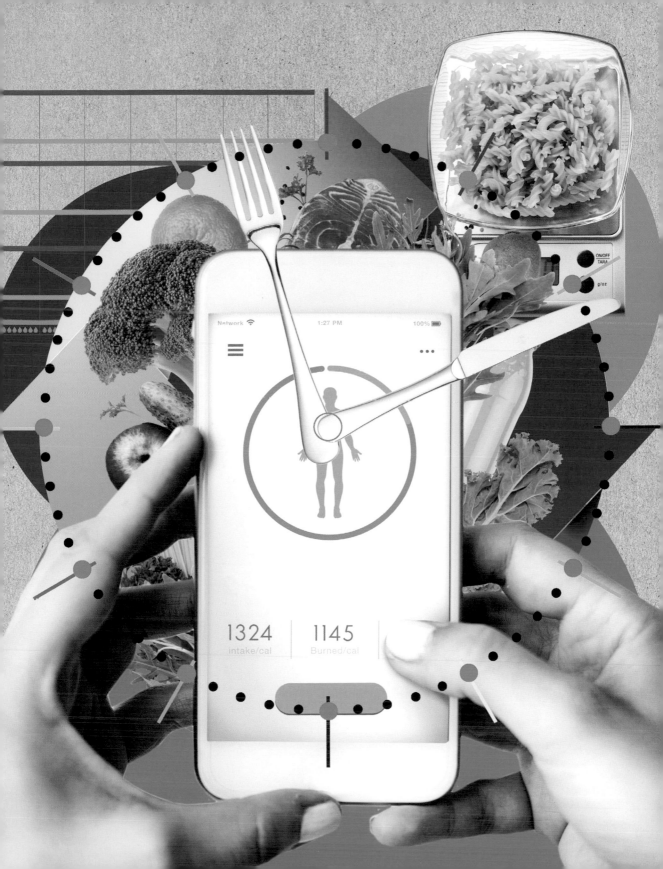

FOODS & HEALTH

allergy Damaging immune response by the body to a substance, such as a food, to which it has become hypersensitive.

amino acids The building blocks of all proteins, amino acids make up a large proportion of cells, muscles and tissue, carrying out many important bodily functions, such as giving cells their structure. Also play a key role in the transport and storage of nutrients. Essential amino acids need to be gained through diet rather than formed by the body itself.

bioactive compounds Extranutritional constituents that typically occur in small quantities in foods. Usually linked with positive effects, and include carotenoids, antioxidants and flavonoids.

bioavailability Extent to which nutrients are digested and absorbed.

cholesterol An animal sterol often classified with dietary fats vital for normal functioning of the body. Mainly made by the liver, but can also be found in some foods. Low density lipoprotein cholesterol (LDL-C) is often referred to as 'bad cholesterol' because too much of it is unhealthy. High density lipoprotein cholesterol (HDL-C) is often referred to as 'good cholesterol' because it is protective. Dietary cholesterol in an egg is not the same as the LDL-C that circulates in blood and blocks arteries, and it is erroneous to believe that dietary cholesterol simply becomes LDL-C once it has been consumed.

coeliac disease Autoimmune disorder from eating gluten, which damages the small intestine. Symptoms include diarrhoea, abdominal pain and bloating.

epidemiology The study of how often diseases occur in different populations and why.

insulin Hormone made by the pancreas that allows your body to use or store glucose from carbohydrates in food for energy. Maintains correct blood sugar level. When cells react abnormally to insulin, this is known as insulin resistance, which increases the risk of developing type 2 diabetes and prediabetes.

gluten Mixture of two proteins, gliadin and glutenin, responsible for the elastic texture of dough.

lactase Enzyme produced by many organisms, located in the small intestine. Essential to the digestion of milk and dairy foods, as it breaks down **lactose**.

lactose Type of sugar mainly found in milk and dairy products.

lipid profile Blood tests that measure levels of lipids (fats and fatty substances, or cholesterols) in the bloodstream. Used as part of a cardiac risk assessment.

mercury Metal found in the environment. Eating a high quantity of foods contaminated with mercury can affect the nervous system and a developing foetus.

micronutrients Vitamins and minerals; required in trace amounts for the healthy functioning of the body.

omega-3 Fatty acids found in fish, especially fatty fish like salmon, tuna, sardine and mackerel. Important for visual and cognitive development and for heart, cognitive and inflammatory health.

polychlorinated biphenyls Manmade industrial chemicals that can be released into the environment through waste and absorbed through the food chain.

probiotic bacteria Live bacteria promoted as having various health benefits, especially for the gut and relating to digestion. Added to yoghurt or taken as supplements.

salmonella Bacteria in contaminated food that causes food poisoning. Symptoms include diarrhoea, stomach cramps, vomiting and fever.

scurvy Severe vitamin C deficiency. Symptoms include fatigue, weakness, severe joint or leg pain, bleeding gums, red or blue spots on the skin, easy bruising.

World Health Organization (WHO) Agency of the United Nations tasked with building a better, healthier future for people all over the world.

FRUIT & VEGETABLES

the 30-second digest

Fruit and vegetables are a major food group and are important components of a healthy diet. Diets rich in fruit and vegetables have been linked to a reduced risk of chronic disease, whereas low fruit and vegetable consumption has been linked to poor health. The World Health Organization (WHO) has stated that, in 2013, an estimated 5.2 million deaths worldwide were attributable to lower than recommended fruit and vegetable consumption. The evidence is strong for cardiovascular disease, relatively consistent for specific cancer sites and is weaker for both diabetes and obesity. Fruit and vegetables are micronutrient- and fibre-rich, as well as containing a range of beneficial non-nutrient components, including plant sterols, flavonoids and other bioactives, which have a range of potential health benefits, including antioxidant and anti-inflammatory properties. Consuming a variety of fruit and vegetables will help to ensure an adequate intake of many of these essential nutrients. Fruit and vegetables are, therefore, recommended across all dietary guidelines. WHO suggests consuming more than 400 grams of fruits and vegetables per day to improve overall health and reduce the risk of certain non-communicable diseases.

RELATED TOPICS
See also
WATER-SOLUBLE VITAMINS
page 28

ORGANIC FOODS
page 142

3-SECOND BIOGRAPHY
JAMES LIND
1716–94
Scottish physician who first demonstrated that scurvy could be remedied by eating citrus fruit.

30-SECOND TEXT
Jayne Woodside

3-SECOND BITE
A high intake of fruits and vegetables has been associated with reduced risk of a number of chronic diseases, including cardiovascular disease in particular.

3-MINUTE SNACK
Although the evidence linking increased fruit and vegetable intake to reduced risk of chronic disease is strong, it is difficult to measure fruit and vegetable intake accurately, and there are some uncertainties regarding the importance of variety, the optimum number of portions and whether different types of fruit and vegetables have different health effects. The effect of storage, processing and cooking methods on nutrient content and therefore health benefits is also uncertain.

Consumption guidelines have been widely translated as five portions of fruit and vegetables per day.

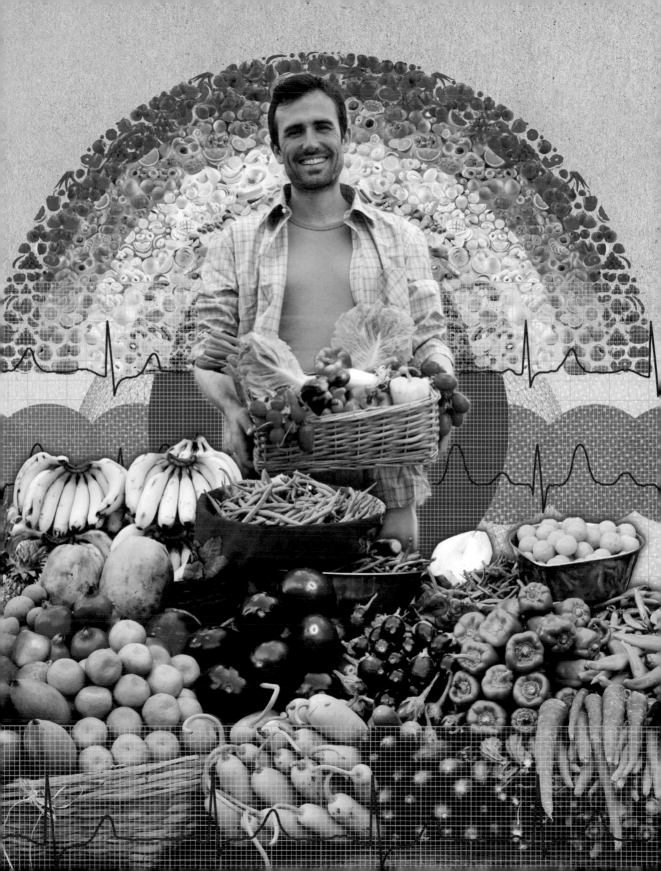

FISH

the 30-second digest

Fish is a very healthy food that may be classed as white fish, fatty fish or shellfish. Fish provides good quality protein and can be a source of many micronutrients, including selenium, iodine and vitamin D. Fish, especially fatty fish like salmon, tuna, sardine and mackerel, is the best source of the omega-3 fatty acids that are important for visual and cognitive development and for heart, cognitive and inflammatory health. Epidemiological studies have shown associations between higher consumption of fish and reduced risk of heart disease, stroke, some cancers, cognitive decline, depression and several other non-communicable diseases. The protective effects of fish are often ascribed to omega-3 fatty acids, but it is likely that the other nutrients in fish also play a role. To obtain sufficient omega-3 fatty acids, it is recommended that people eat one or two servings of fatty fish each week. In many countries, fish consumption, especially of fatty fish, is lower than recommended. Despite its clear health benefits, fish can be a source of toxins such as mercury and contaminants such as polychlorinated biphenyls, which are harmful to health. These compounds can become concentrated within the marine food chain. For this reason, pregnant women are advised not to eat certain fish.

RELATED TOPICS
See also
FATS
page 22

DIETARY FATS &
HEART DISEASE
page 98

OMEGA-3 FATTY ACIDS
page 122

3-SECOND BITE
Fish is a good source of micronutrients and of omega-3 fatty acids. Yet, in many countries, people eat less fish than recommended.

3-MINUTE SNACK
Commercial fishing is a major global industry. It can have an adverse impact on fish stocks and the environment, and it is likely that fishing in its current form is unsustainable in some locations. Since fish are an important source of protein, micronutrients and omega-3 fatty acids, the lack of sustainability of fishing is a challenge to human health and well-being. Fish farming is only a partial solution.

3-SECOND BIOGRAPHY
MASAZUMI HARADA
1934–2012
Japanese doctor and medical researcher who worked on the effects of Minamata disease, a severe mercury poisoning that occurred in Minamata, Japan, during the 1950s and 60s, as a result of a petrochemical company discharging heavy metal waste into the sea.

30-SECOND TEXT
Philip C Calder

Low in fat, shellfish are a source of omega-3, protein, iron, zinc, copper and vitamin B_{12}.

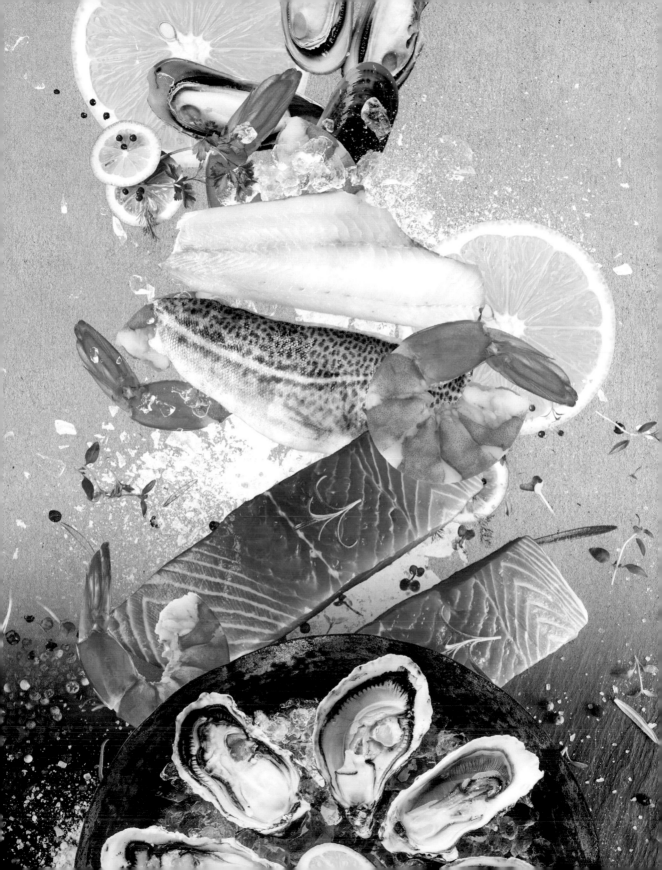

MILK & DAIRY

the 30-second digest

Dairy foods are not essential in our diet, but can contribute to over 40% of daily intake of calcium, iodine, phosphorus and some B-vitamins in Europe and the USA. Dairy also provides a higher quality of protein than meat. All dairy foods are made from milk that comes from ruminant animals such as cows, sheep, goats and water buffalo and have been consumed for over 7,500 years in some European populations. There is a misconception that milk is a high-fat food, yet whole milk contains only 3.6% fat, semi-skimmed 1.7% and skimmed 0%. Dairy foods are the main contributor to saturated fat intake in many countries, but a high intake of dairy (excluding butter and cream) is not generally associated with heart disease risk. On the contrary, proteins, calcium, magnesium and probiotic bacteria in dairy foods have been linked to some beneficial effects on heart health, including lowering blood pressure. While some individuals develop an allergy to milk protein, others have lactose intolerance and are unable to digest dairy sugar (lactose). Interestingly, adult lactose intolerance is a normal condition in mammals. However, most humans have a genetic mutation that enables them to consume dairy products in adulthood, due to the persistence of lactase, required for lactose digestion.

RELATED TOPICS
See also
FOOD ALLERGIES & INTOLERANCES
page 100

VITAMIN D & CALCIUM
page 126

PROBIOTICS & PREBIOTICS
page 128

3-SECOND BITE
Milk is a highly nutritious food, with high absorbable calcium for bone health, yet humans are the only animals to drink milk throughout life.

3-MINUTE SNACK
Milk is an excellent medium for bacterial growth, so to prolong its shelf life and ensure it is safe to drink, milk can be heat-treated by pasteurization. This process involves heating milk to 72°C (162°F) for 15–21 seconds, which maintains its nutritive content, apart from a small loss of vitamin B_{12}. In the production of cheese and yoghurt, added bacteria ferment lactose, producing lactic acid, which thickens the milk and gives cheese and yoghurt their characteristic sour taste.

3-SECOND BIOGRAPHY
LOUIS PASTEUR
1822–95
French microbiologist who was the first to conduct pasteurization tests in 1862 for milk preservation; credited with revolutionizing the safety of milk, enabling it to be stored and distributed widely.

30-SECOND TEXT
Julie A Lovegrove

The commercial pasteurization of milk was introduced in 1895, and modern methods are controlled by food safety agencies.

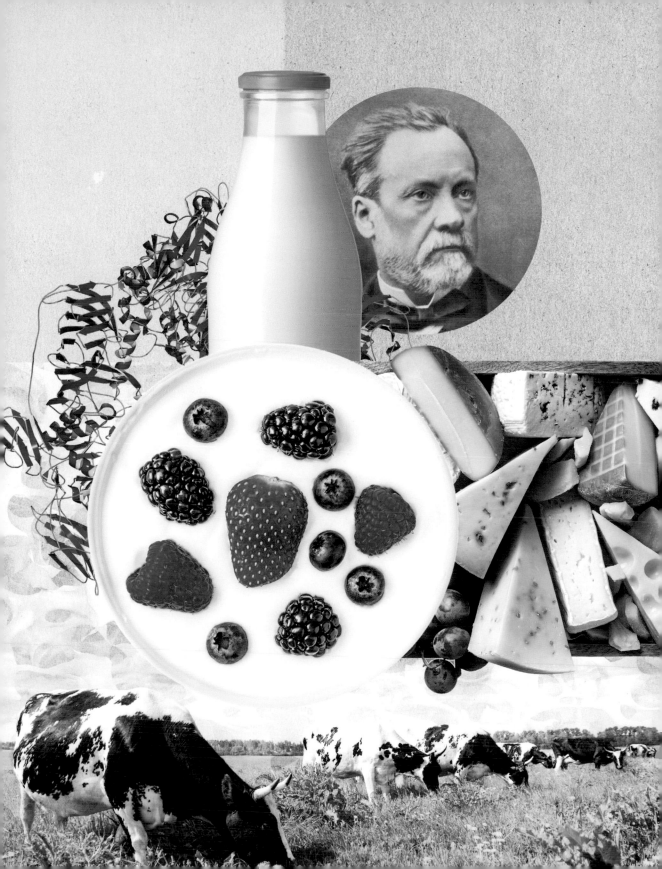

EGGS

the 30-second digest

Egg yolk contains all of the essential ingredients to build a living organism and provides a richer source of micronutrients than any other single food. Egg white contains protein that is superior to beef steak in nutritional quality (content of essential amino acids) and bioavailability. Eggs also boast the highest ratio of nutrient to energy density than any other food. So why have dietary guidelines restricted the intake of such a nutritious food? An egg yolk provides the main source of dietary cholesterol (approximately 200 mg/egg), which has been linked to coronary heart disease (CHD) by its association with 'low density lipoprotein cholesterol' (LDL-C). However, the dietary cholesterol in an egg is not the same as the LDL cholesterol that circulates in our blood and blocks arteries, and it is erroneous to believe that dietary cholesterol simply becomes LDL cholesterol in blood once it has been eaten. Eating an excessive amount of dietary cholesterol in eggs can increase blood LDL-cholesterol – by reducing the ability of our cells to extract LDL-C from the blood – but for most healthy people, an egg a day will have no significant effect in raising LDL-cholesterol, or risk of CHD, especially in comparison to the effects of eating too much saturated fat and being overweight.

There is no such thing as a 'superfood' for improving human health. But if there were, the egg must qualify as a major contender.

3-MINUTE SNACK

Eggs have always courted controversy, with fears over the impact of their cholesterol on CHD, allergy in response to their protein and the risk of salmonella infection, which is now mostly eradicated by mass vaccination programmes. Nevertheless, the egg prevails as a highly popular and versatile food that is unmatched in its capacity to nourish humans throughout their life course.

RELATED TOPICS

See also
FATS
page 22

DIETARY FATS &
HEART DISEASE
page 98

FREE-RANGE & INTENSIVELY
FARMED FOODS
page 144

3-SECOND BIOGRAPHIES
DR ANCEL KEYS
1904–2004
Keys stated that there was no evidence from studies in humans to support the idea that the amount of cholesterol in the diet can influence the level of blood cholesterol.

JOSEPH GOLDSTEIN &
MICHAEL BROWN
1940– & 1941–
Discovered the LDL receptor pathway as the mechanism that regulates cholesterol metabolism.

30-SECOND TEXT
Bruce A Griffin

A deepening knowledge of cholesterol has led to the relaxation of restrictions on eggs.

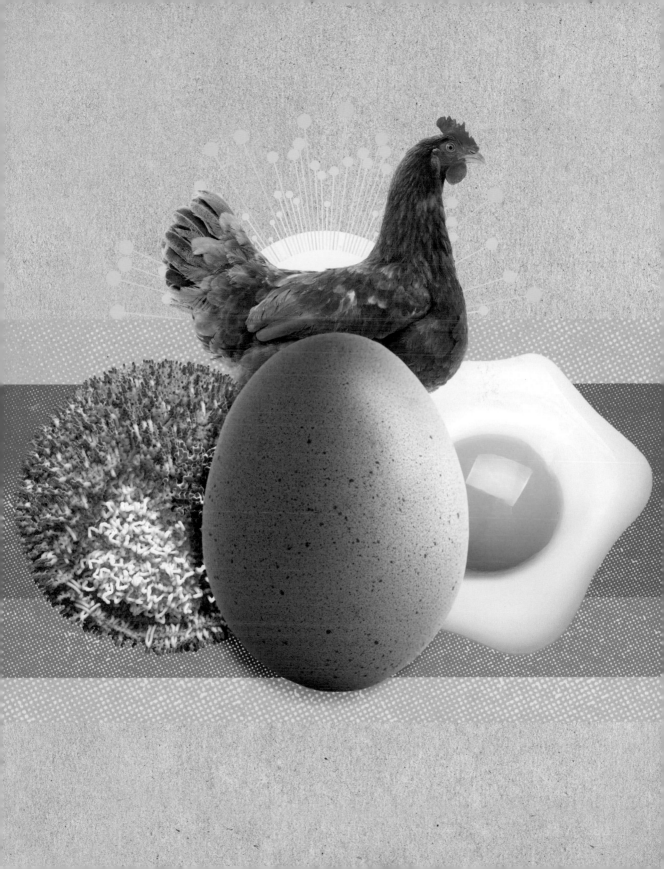

NUTS

the 30-second digest

There has been increasing interest in nuts and how they might improve human health. Peanuts and tree nuts are foods that most commonly cause an allergic reaction, but it has been demonstrated that consumption of a frequent peanut-containing snack by infants who are at high-risk of developing a peanut allergy may prevent the development of allergy. Nuts are a varied food group, including, for example, tree nuts (almonds, hazelnuts, walnuts, pistachios, Brazil nuts and cashews) and legume seeds (peanuts). Nuts are nutrient-dense foods that are high in energy, but also with a favourable fatty acid (FA) profile (high in monounsaturated FAs and/or polyunsaturated FAs) and contain a range of bioactive compounds that also have proposed health benefits, such as vitamins, minerals and other antioxidants. Increasing nut intake has been demonstrated to reduce blood pressure, improve regulation of glucose, improve blood vessel health, reduce inflammation and improve lipid profile. Therefore, increasing intake could reduce risk of heart disease, and nuts are a key food group consumed within a Mediterranean Diet, which has been proven to be heart-healthy. Nuts have a high energy content, but concerns about them being fattening are largely unfounded.

3-SECOND BITE
Eating more nuts will not cause weight gain, can improve other risk factors for heart disease and is part of an overall healthy diet pattern.

3-MINUTE SNACK
Nuts are thought to reduce the risk of heart disease. Whether different types of nuts have different health effects is not yet well studied, so mixed nuts – unsalted and unroasted – are recommended. People with poor dental health may report difficulties eating nuts, and therefore the form of nuts consumed (such as ground or sliced) needs to be considered in some population groups.

RELATED TOPICS
See also
PROTEIN
page 16

MEDITERRANEAN DIET
page 68

FOOD ALLERGIES & INTOLERANCES
page 100

3-SECOND BIOGRAPHY
GIDEON LACK
Lead investigator on the LEAP study, which was the first randomized trial to prevent peanut allergy in a large cohort of high-risk infants.

30-SECOND TEXT
Jayne Woodside

Increased consumption does not necessarily lead to weight gain, and nuts can increase satiety.

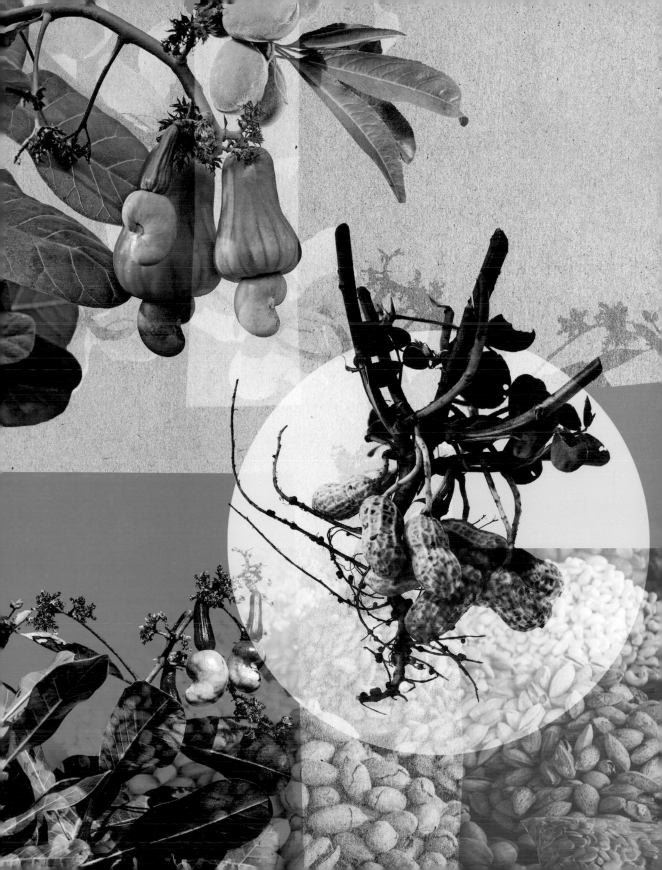

GRAINS & GLUTEN

the 30-second digest

The edible seeds from plants of the grass family are called 'cereal grains', or 'cereals'. The general term for both the fruit (the seed or kernel) and the plant is 'grain'. Major grain types worldwide are wheat, rice, corn (maize), barley, sorghum, oats, rye and millet. Other important plants that are used as grains but are not technically grains include wild rice, buckwheat, amaranth and quinoa. Wheat flour is the preferred flour for baking due to the formation of gluten when the flour is mixed with water and stirred or beaten, such as when making a batter or kneading a dough. Gluten, a mixture of two proteins, gliadin and glutenin, is responsible for the elastic texture of dough. Besides wheat, gluten can also be found in barley, rye and triticale. It gives baked goods soft, fluffy and moist qualities. Without it, bread would lose its shape, dry out and quickly become stale. However, individuals with coeliac disease (an autoimmune disorder that damages the small intestine), wheat allergy (allergic reactions caused by gluten or other wheat protein) or non-coeliac gluten sensitivity eat naturally gluten-free diets or products made with gluten-free flours, such as those from corn, rice, potato and soy, amongst others.

RELATED TOPICS

See also
FOOD ALLERGIES &
INTOLERANCES
page 100

REFINING
page 136

3-SECOND BITE

Gluten refers to proteins found in wheat, barley, rye and triticale, providing baked products with texture, moisture and flavour; however, it can cause an immune-mediated reaction in the small intestine.

3-MINUTE SNACK

Gluten-free diets are popular, and can benefit those who experience adverse reactions and/or suffer from related conditions such as coeliac disease, wheat allergy or non-coeliac gluten sensitivity. However, there is little clinical evidence to support the claim that a gluten-free diet is a 'healthier' diet directly related to improved health, weight loss or increased energy.

3-SECOND BIOGRAPHY
WILLEM-KAREL DICKE
1905–62
Dutch paediatrician who was the first to develop a gluten-free diet for the treatment of coeliac disease.

30-SECOND TEXT
Zhiping Yu

Corn is from a different branch of the grain family than the gluten grains of wheat, barley and rye.

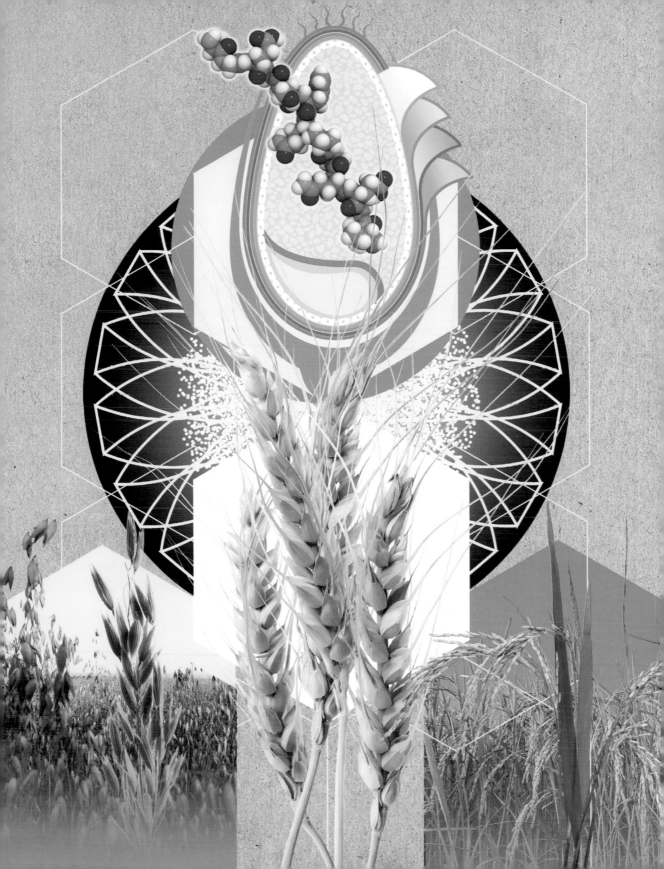

VEGAN & VEGETARIANISM

the 30-second digest

Between 1 and 10% of the population in developed countries follow a vegetarian diet. Many individuals and special interest groups claim that vegetarian diets can prolong life and promote health and vitality. These claims are largely unsubstantiated in terms of reliable scientific evidence. However, populations following vegetarian diets do seem to have reduced risk of heart disease and obesity. It is widely recognized, however, that over-reliance on one single food or food group will not provide the range of nutrients required for optimum health and well-being. If a particular food or food group is not consumed routinely, alternative nutrient sources must be included; for example, instead of meat, plant-based protein sources such as legumes. Very restrictive or unbalanced vegetarian diets can result in nutrient deficiencies, particularly iron, calcium, zinc and vitamins B_{12} and D. This is especially the case for groups at risk of nutrient deficiency, including infants, children, menstruating and lactating women and athletes. Vegetarian and vegan diets can, however, be balanced and healthy for all stages of life, provided appropriate preparation and planning are followed. Vegans may require supplementation if adequate intake of nutrients cannot be achieved.

3-SECOND BITE
Following a well-balanced and varied vegetarian or vegan diet may be associated with improved health outcomes, especially for heart disease and obesity.

3-MINUTE SNACK
Whilst vegetarian and vegan diets are potentially beneficial to health, if they are well-balanced and varied, such diet patterns are highly heterogeneous in nature, which makes thorough assessment of their effects on health difficult. Furthermore, vegetarian lifestyles often encompass other health behaviours which can improve health, for example, being physically active, not smoking and limiting alcohol consumption; therefore, the effect of the dietary pattern *per se* is difficult to determine.

RELATED TOPICS
See also
FRUIT & VEGETABLES
page 54

BABIES, INFANTS & CHILDREN
page 76

RED & PROCESSED MEATS
page 110

3-SECOND BIOGRAPHY
PYTHAGORAS
c. 570 BCE
Greek philosopher and mathematician who promoted benevolence among all species and followed what could be described as a vegetarian diet.

30-SECOND TEXT
Jayne Woodside

Any restrictive diet requires some rebalancing of food types and nutrients, for optimum health.

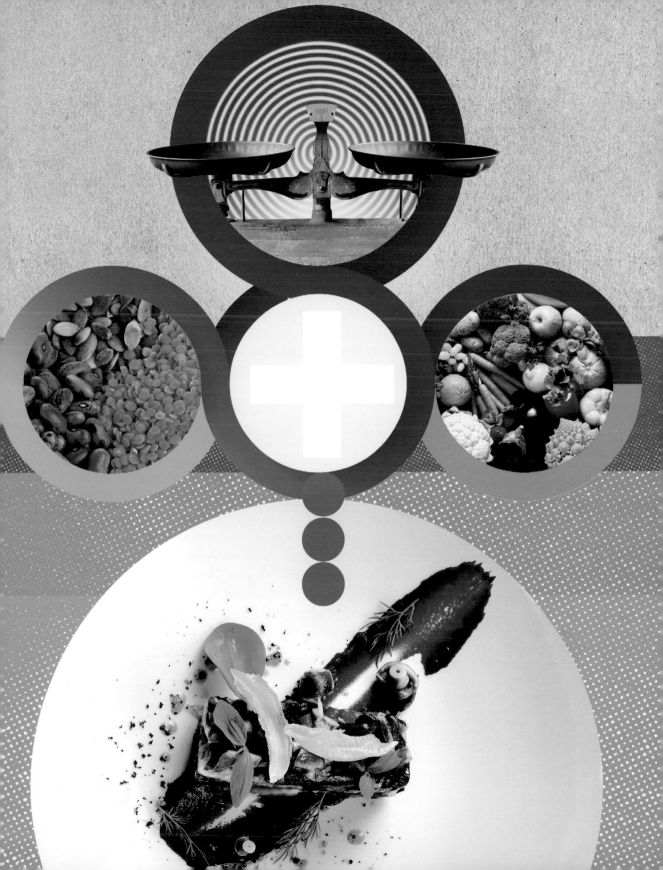

MEDITERRANEAN DIET

the 30-second digest

3-SECOND BITE
Changing to a
Mediterranean Diet
pattern is likely to reduce
risk of heart disease and
may benefit a range of
chronic diseases.

3-MINUTE SNACK
The Mediterranean Diet
has been proposed as an
alternative and palatable
lifestyle change that is
beneficial to health. What
is not yet clear is whether
non-Mediterranean
populations can adopt
and maintain dietary
behaviours consistent with
a traditional Mediterranean
diet – because of the
required changes in foods
consumed, eating patterns
and food culture – and
there are concerns that
Mediterranean populations
are changing their diet
habits towards a
Western-style diet.

The Mediterranean Diet is a diet pattern rich in fruit, vegetables, legumes, nuts, fish and olive oil, and low in red meat and processed foods. There has always been regional variation and, more recently, changes over time in the exact foods and how frequently they are consumed, but the traditional pattern is based on the typical diet of many regions in Greece and southern Italy in the early 1960s. The Mediterranean Diet has been rated as the dietary pattern most likely, based on current knowledge, to offer protection against cardiovascular disease. This is supported by robust and consistent evidence from different types of population studies, including trials where people have changed their diet and rates of heart disease have been reduced. How the diet protects the heart is not fully understood, but those who follow it more closely seem to have a healthier lipid profile, lower blood pressure, lower insulin resistance and less inflammation. Emerging evidence also suggests that following a Mediterranean Diet may have additional benefits for overall longevity and other chronic diseases, such as diabetes, cancer and Alzheimer's disease. The health benefits offered appear to be attributable to interactions between different food components rather than the effects of single nutrients.

RELATED TOPICS
See also
FRUIT & VEGETABLES
page 54

FISH
page 56

DIETARY FATS &
HEART DISEASE
page 98

3-SECOND BIOGRAPHIES
ANCEL KEYS
1904–2004
American physiologist
who explored whether
differences in diet could
explain differences in rates
of heart disease.

MICHEL DELORGERIL
1950–
French cardiologist who was
the first to demonstrate that
heart disease patients who
adhered to a Mediterranean
Diet reduced their chances
of a further heart attack.

30-SECOND TEXT
Jayne Woodside

There are concerns that the modern-day Mediterranean diet is losing its unique components.

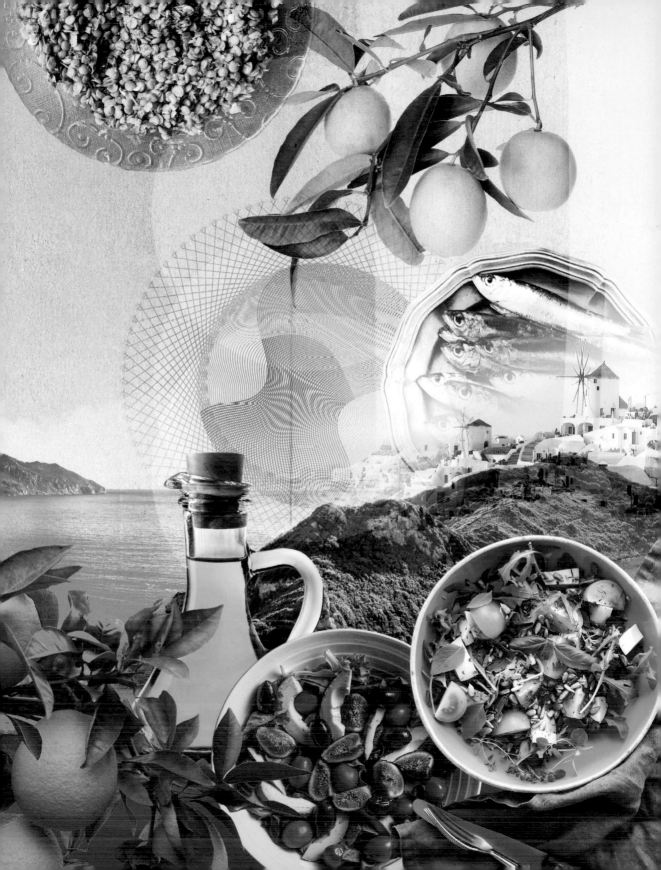

26 January 1904
Born in Colorado Springs, USA

1930
First PhD in Oceanography and Biology, UC Berkeley

1935
Appointed Director of the International High Altitude Expedition to Chile

1936
Awarded second PhD in Physiology, King's College, Cambridge

1937
Founds the Laboratory of Physiological Hygiene at the University of Minnesota

1941
Develops pocket-sized 'K-rations' for the US military in WWII

1944
Initiates the Minnesota Starvation Experiment

1947
Initiates the Minnesota Business and Professional Men's Study

1950
Appointed Chair of the World Health Organization's first Joint Commission on Food & Agriculture, Rome

1954
Establishes cardiovascular epidemiology as a new discipline

1961
Nicknamed 'Mr Cholesterol' on the front page of *Time* magazine

1970
First publication of Seven Countries Study results

1980
Publishes third book with co-author wife – *Eat Well, Live Well*

20 November 2004
Dies in Minnesota, USA, at the age of 100

ANCEL KEYS

Ancel Keys was a physiologist and pioneer in cardiovascular epidemiology, who established that a high intake of saturated fat increases the risk of coronary heart disease (CHD) by raising the level of blood cholesterol. This discovery became known as the 'diet-heart hypothesis' and has been the cornerstone of dietary guidelines to prevent CHD since the early 1980s.

Keys was a gifted and inquisitive child, but a wayward teenager who had a series of menial labouring jobs. He returned to higher education in his late twenties, when he gained two doctorates and a reputation for applying mathematics to quantify biological phenomena. Keys' first experience of fame was when he founded the pocket-sized military 'K-ration' (an emergency, mobile source of food that could provide soldiers with enough energy in the field for two weeks), before turning his attention at the end of the war to the effects of starvation and how to rehabilitate malnourished post-war survivors. This led to his curiosity over the variation in incidence of CHD in different countries, especially the low prevalence of CHD in underfed European populations, contrasted with a high prevalence of CHD in affluent American businessmen. Keys was also fascinated by the increased rate of CHD in Japanese immigrants to the US who adopted a Westernized diet, and suggested that all of these observations could be explained by a high intake of saturated fat raising the level of blood cholesterol. This theory was supported by his landmark Seven Countries Study, in which a high incidence of death from CHD in men in Finland and the USA was contrasted with the low incidence of CHD in Italy, Greece and Japan. The results from this study were used to formulate the 'Keys equations' for predicting the opposing effects of dietary saturated and polyunsaturated fats on blood cholesterol, which are still used in clinical practice today.

Ancel Keys was an advocate for the benefits of the Mediterranean diet in preventing CHD, long before the impact of this diet was formally tested and shown to prevent death from CHD in a randomly controlled trial called 'PREDIMED' in 2006. While Keys' contribution to nutritional science has had an incalculable impact in preventing death from premature CHD, there have been allegations that he manipulated his results to concoct his theory about saturated fat and CHD. Keys died before he could defend himself against these allegations, but, fortunately, his reputation and monumental contribution to nutrition science have been redeemed by those who worked closely with him, in a White Paper commissioned by The True Health Initiative in 2017.

Bruce A Griffin

A LIFETIME OF NUTRITION

adolescence Mental and cultural transition from childhood to adulthood; overlaps with **puberty**.

anaemia Develops when the blood does not contain enough healthy red blood cells or haemoglobin, important for carrying oxygen around the body. There are many types and causes, including iron deficiency. Symptoms include lethargy, shortness of breath, pale complexion and dry nails.

bariatric surgery Weight-loss surgery, which might be recommended for very obese people (BMI of over 35). Could include placement of a gastric band around the stomach, a gastric bypass to join the top part of the stomach to the small intestine, or a sleeve gastrectomy, in which some of the stomach is removed.

bifidobacteria Major type of bacteria that make up the gut microbiome. Some bifidobacteria are used as probiotics. Found in foods such as live-culture yoghurt.

dementia Syndrome associated with an ongoing decline of brain functioning. Can affect memory, thinking speed, language, understanding, judgement, mood and movement.

folate Also known as vitamin B9. Folate in the form of folic acid is advised for pregnant women (to prevent neural tube defects in the developing foetus) and to prevent a type of **anaemia**. Essential for DNA synthesis and metabolizing amino acids, it is an essential vitamin.

lactation Secretion of milk from the mammary glands; when a mother feeds her baby. Suckling by the baby to the mother's breast stimulates the supply of milk, which provides essential nutrients and an array of bioactive substances absorbed by the infant for brain, immune and gut development.

malnutrition When a person doesn't eat enough, through illness, or when there is insufficient amounts or quality of food, resulting in insufficient essential nutrients. The consequence is reduced growth or weight loss. Symptoms can include a lack of interest in eating and drinking, chronic fatigue, feeling weak and a diminished immune system.

menopause When women stop menstruating and being able to conceive. Occurs between 45 and 55 years of age, as a woman's **oestrogen** and **progesterone** levels decline, and typically lasts for four years. Symptoms include hot flushes, vaginal dryness, trouble sleeping and mood changes.

micronutrients Vitamins and minerals; required in trace amounts for the healthy functioning of the body.

obesity Significantly overweight, with excess body fat; commonly measured using BMI (body mass index). Generally caused when more calories – particularly those in fatty and sugary foods – are consumed than burned (through physical activity). The excess energy is stored by the body as fat. Can lead to diabetes, heart disease, cancer, stroke and depression.

oestrogen Primary female sex hormone. Secreted by the ovaries, it plays a key role in **puberty**, the menstrual cycle and sex drive, and even in cognition, mental health and binge eating. Declines after **menopause**.

osteoporosis Bone-weakening condition that develops over several years until a fall or impact can cause a bone fracture. Postmenopausal women are at risk. A healthy diet (including foods rich in calcium and vitamin D), regular exercise and reducing alcohol consumption can help prevent the condition.

pathogens Micro-organisms, such as bacteria and viruses, that cause disease.

Bacteria release toxins, and viruses damage cells. White blood cells can ingest and destroy pathogens, which can be consumed through contaminated food or drinks, resulting in flu-like symptoms and nausea, vomiting, diarrhoea or fever.

progesterone Female sex hormones produced by the ovaries and adrenal glands. Plays an important role in sustaining pregnancy and regulating the menstrual cycle. High levels are thought to be responsible for symptoms of PMS (Pre-Menstrual Syndrome).

puberty Physical changes that mature a child's body into an adult's body capable of sexual reproduction. The brain sends hormonal signals to the gonads – ovaries in girls, testes in boys. The average age for girls to start this process is 11; for boys it's 12, and it typically takes four years. See also **Adolescence**.

sarcopenia Disease associated with the ageing process. Loss of muscle mass and strength affects balance, gait and ability to perform daily tasks.

type 2 diabetes Llifelong condition that causes the level of sugar (glucose) in the blood to become too high, as a result of the insufficient production of insulin or the insulin being ineffective.

BABIES, INFANTS & CHILDREN

the 30-second digest

3-SECOND BITE
Children are not little adults – give them plenty of fruit, vegetables, high quality proteins and wholegrain carbs. Go easy on the sugar and salt to keep them healthy.

3-MINUTE SNACK
It's vital to get children's diets right. Firstly, early eating habits track into adulthood, so a healthy start will have a positive lifelong influence on food choice. Secondly, as diseases such as heart disease and type 2 diabetes have their origins in adolescence, a balanced diet can help prevent future illness.

The first 24 months of life are a time of rapid growth and development. After this, growth slows, but mental and social development continues apace. This is why infants and children need good quality protein and sufficient vitamins and minerals to meet their needs. Proteins support growth and development, especially muscle and bones. Fibre is needed for digestive function and to prevent constipation, and can be found in fruit, vegetables and wholegrains. Calcium and vitamin D are vital for optimal bone health, as bone density increases until its peak in young adulthood. Iron is vital for red blood cells, which carry oxygen around the body. Studies show that young children and teenage girls have a higher risk of low iron status, which can impact on immune function and cognitive development. Due to high nutritional needs and the fact that fussy eating is common, several countries recommend supplementation with vitamins A, C and D from infanthood until school-age. A fish oil supplement is useful if your child won't eat oily fish. As children's diets can influence future food preferences, and teeth are susceptible to decay, sugary foods and drinks should be limited. Salt should not be added to babies' and toddlers' meals as their underdeveloped kidneys cannot process the extra sodium.

RELATED TOPICS
See also
PROTEIN
page 16

FAT-SOLUBLE VITAMINS
page 26

MILK & DAIRY
page 58

3-SECOND BIOGRAPHIES
JANE WARDLE
1950–2015
British health psychologist who published influential work on children's eating behaviour and how it relates to risk of obesity.

MARIA MAKRIDES
Australian researcher who showed the importance of omega-3 fatty acids to the infant brain.

LEANN BIRCH
American professor who demonstrated that young children are uniquely able to match their calorie intakes to requirements.

30-SECOND TEXT
Carrie Ruxton

Fresh fruit and vegetables can be introduced when a baby starts weaning.

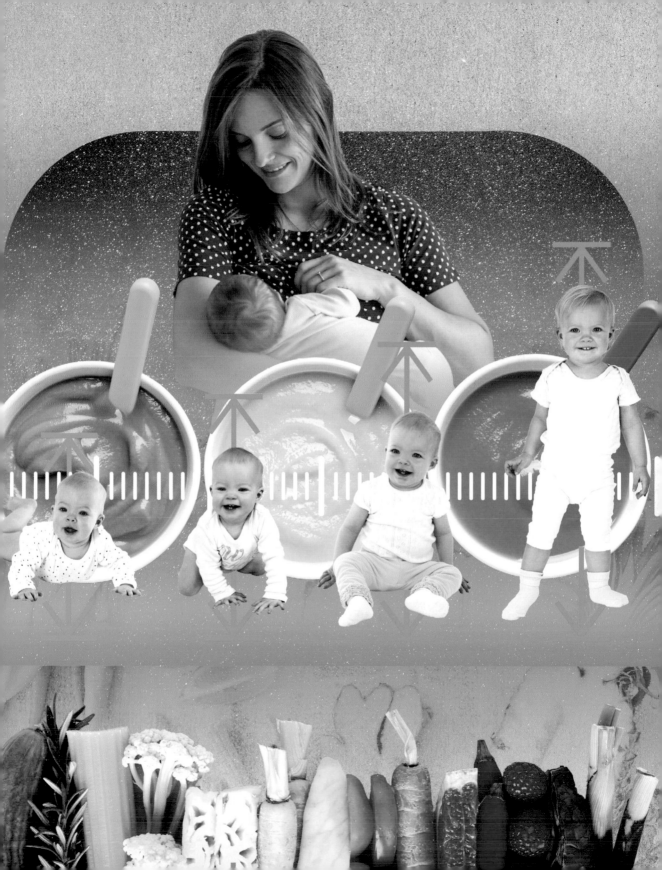

ADOLESCENTS

the 30-second digest

3-SECOND BITE
Adolescence is a period of significant growth and change in which good nutrition can play a key role in overall health.

3-MINUTE SNACK
Appropriate parental involvement in healthy eating is vital during adolescence. It's important to provide opportunities where teens can make their own eating choices, but also foster a positive, supportive environment around healthy foods such as fresh produce, high-fibre foods and proteins. Teens should be encouraged to drink water rather than sweetened beverages, as well as to take regular physical activity.

Adolescence is the period of growth and development that occurs during the ages of 10 to 19. This period is characterized by physical changes, known as puberty, as well as social and emotional changes. The most common and visible changes of puberty are related to sexual maturation, which begins between ages 9 and 13 in girls and 11-and-a-half and 12 years in boys. Both genders will also experience significant growth in height and bone mass during this time period. Due to all these changes in a child's physical appearance, a greater self-awareness is often developed, and the child may be self-conscious for the first time. Relationships are also shifting as greater significance is placed on a child's social relationships and less on their family relationships. An adolescent might also want to exert more independence in making their own food choices. This presents a potential risk for choosing too many sugary and fat-dense foods while not eating enough fresh produce and high-fibre foods. The prevalence of adolescents being overweight or obese has significantly increased in recent years and these factors are one of the underlying reasons. Other nutrition-related concerns include adequate iron, vitamin D and calcium.

RELATED TOPICS
See also
MINERALS
page 24

OVERWEIGHT & OBESITY
page 86

VITAMIN D & CALCIUM
page 126

3-SECOND BIOGRAPHY
G STANLEY HALL
1846–1924
American psychologist and educator who was the originator of the study of adolescence with his seminal work *Adolescence*, published in 1904.

30-SECOND TEXT
Jenna Braddock

Adolescence is an important life stage for kids to begin healthy habits that will serve them well the rest of their life.

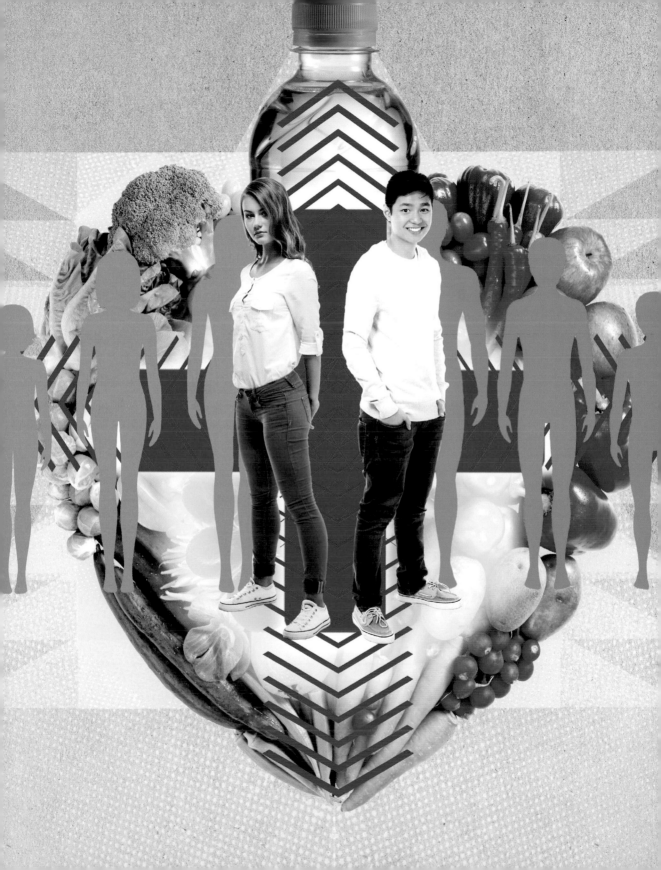

PREGNANCY & LACTATION

the 30-second digest

During pregnancy, maternal physiology undergoes dramatic changes to support the developing foetus. Changes include increases in blood volume and the size and function of major organs (heart, kidneys, pituitary, thyroid, mammaries and uterus). Maternal nutrient intake needs to support these changes as well as the developing child. Surprisingly, the additional energy requirements (above those for a non-pregnant woman) are not substantial, estimated at about a further 10% during the last three months of pregnancy. Excessive calories before and during pregnancy are associated with adverse outcomes for both mother and baby and are a major concern for many populations. An appropriate supply of micronutrients is important for successful pregnancy and lactation. During pregnancy, the tissue development of mother and baby requires a range of micronutrients, including those involved in cell, red blood cell and DNA synthesis, such as folate and iron. The multiple roles of micronutrients in the developing foetus are complex, and an adequate supply during – and for some nutrients (such as folate) before – pregnancy is important. Micronutrient requirements are partly dependent on the population and setting, which determine the maternal status.

RELATED TOPICS
See also
FAT-SOLUBLE VITAMINS
page 26

WATER-SOLUBLE VITAMINS
page 28

BABIES, INFANTS & CHILDREN
page 76

3-SECOND BIOGRAPHY
DAVID BARKER
1938–2013
British Professor who first proposed the theory of 'Developmental Origins of Health and Disease' or 'foetal programming', suggesting that the early life environment of the foetus influenced lifelong patterns of health and disease.

30-SECOND TEXT
Philip C Calder &
Elizabeth A Miles

3-SECOND BITE
Eating for two? Optimal nutrition during pregnancy needs to support the maternal physiological changes required to ensure successful pregnancy, foetal development and lactation.

3-MINUTE SNACK
Nutritional support of pregnancy is not just a nine-month concern. It benefits the mother and ensures a healthier neonate, but has implications far beyond this. David Barker first published the idea that influences on early life development had lifelong consequences for offspring. He showed that having a low birth weight led to greater risk of dying from coronary heart disease before the age of 65 years.

Optimal nutrient status is key to maintaining maternal health and providing short- and long-term health to the child.

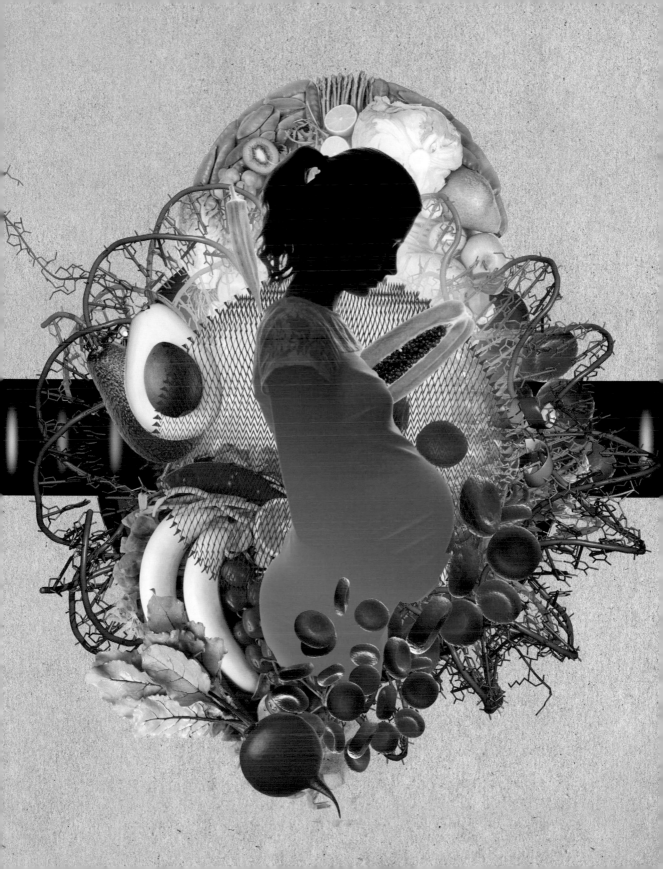

POSTMENOPAUSAL WOMEN

the 30-second digest

A postmenopausal woman has ended her reproductive years, which is usually in her late 40s or early 50s. This ageing process occurs as the ovaries no longer produce sufficient levels of oestrogen and progesterone, causing the ovaries to stop releasing eggs. During menopause, oestrogen levels decline, metabolism decreases and weight gain due to poor dietary and lifestyle choices are at their peak. Common menopausal symptoms, such as hot flushes, night sweats and increased irritability, may fade during the postmenopausal period. During post-menopause, when oestrogen levels are significantly lower, women have an increased risk of heart disease and osteoporosis. Heart disease is one of the leading causes of death in postmenopausal women due to increased body fat accumulation, the ageing process and changes in glucose metabolism. Consuming a heart-healthy diet which is rich in fruits, vegetables, legumes, whole grains and nuts may result in positive benefits. Osteoporosis may also occur as a result of reduced calcium, vitamin D and protein intake, along with low levels of physical activity. To strengthen bones, it is important to consume calcium and vitamin D. Rich sources of vitamin D include fatty fish and egg yolks; rich sources of calcium include dairy and kale.

3-SECOND BITE
Postmenopausal women suffer from a decrease in oestrogen production, affecting mineral absorption and ultimately increasing risk of heart disease and osteoporosis.

3-MINUTE SNACK
Women can boost their diet with increased consumption of healthy foods, such as fruits, vegetables, legumes, whole grains and nuts, to decrease risk of heart disease and osteoporosis. Adding daily physical activity can also help to increase heart and bone strength. Including both aerobic exercises (walking, running, cycling) and strength training exercises (lifting weights, body weight exercises) can contribute to an overall healthy lifestyle.

RELATED TOPICS
See also
FRUIT & VEGETABLES
page 54

DIETARY FATS &
HEART DISEASE
page 98

VITAMIN D & CALCIUM
page 126

3-SECOND BIOGRAPHIES
ADOLF BUTENANDT &
EDWARD ADELBERT DOISY
1903–95 & 1893–1986
German and American biochemists (respectively) who both independently discovered oestrogen; however, only Butenandt was awarded a Nobel Prize in Chemistry.

30-SECOND TEXT
Kristen Hicks-Roof

Balanced nutrition and daily exercise are vital components of a comprehensive health programme.

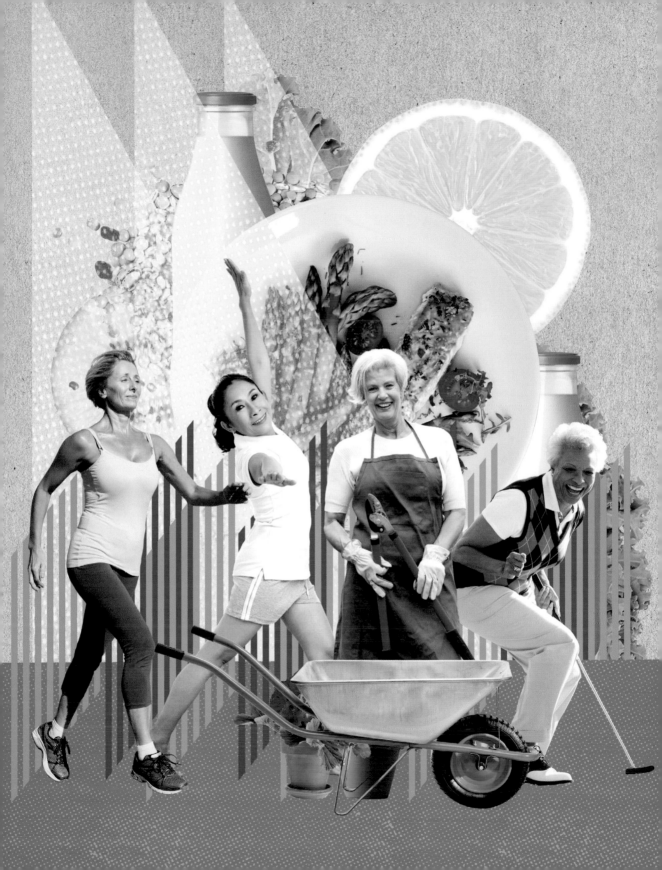

THE ELDERLY

the 30-second digest

Ageing brings changes that

impact on dietary needs as well as health. Muscle mass is harder to build and maintain, leading to the wasting condition sarcopenia. Nutrient absorption is reduced, especially for vitamin B12, folic acid, calcium, zinc and magnesium. Skin synthesis of vitamin D in response to sunlight also tails off. Another important change is to gut bacteria: in young people, these are diverse and skewed towards 'friendly' species such as bifidobacteria; in the elderly, both diversity and friendly species reduce, creating ideal conditions for pathogens. To keep healthy, elderly people should aim for a high-protein, high-fibre diet that includes nutrient-rich lean meat, poultry, eggs, oily fish and nuts, as well as fruit and vegetables, which are high in antioxidants such as vitamin A and C. Portions can be small and frequent to overcome reduced appetite. Soft foods are useful where dental problems exist. Supplements of calcium and vitamin D have been shown to help maintain bone density and prevent falls, probably through improved muscle function, while omega-3 fatty acids (from oily fish or fish oil supplements) have been linked to a reduced risk of dementia-type conditions. Additional B vitamins may help to slow cognitive decline.

RELATED TOPICS
See also
PROTEIN
page 16

FIBRE
page 20

OMGEA-3 FATTY ACIDS
page 122

3-SECOND BIOGRAPHIES
WILLIAM BOSWORTH CASTLE
1897–1990
American physician who discovered the gastric intrinsic factor, the absence of which causes pernicious anaemia, particularly in the elderly.

MARTHA CLARE MORRIS
1955–
American epidemiologist who developed important research linking oily fish consumption to reduced dementia risk.

30-SECOND TEXT
Carrie Ruxton

3-SECOND BITE
Healthier ageing can be achieved by choosing nutrient-rich, high-fibre foods and eating protein-containing foods two to three times a day.

3-MINUTE SNACK
An ageing population, coupled with unhealthy Western diets and lifestyles, means that the average person will spend around a fifth of their lifetime in poor health. A better quality of life in old age requires a shift from low-fibre, high saturated-fat diets packed with processed foods towards nutrient-rich, high-fibre diets, making every calorie count.

Studies show that diet can help to slow the impact of ageing, leading to a better quality of life.

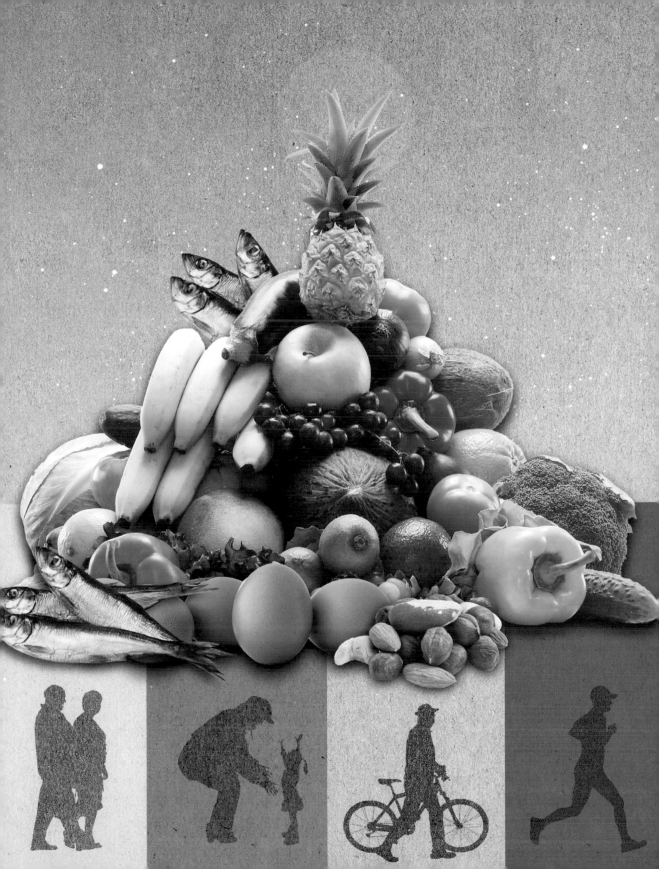

OVERWEIGHT & OBESITY

the 30-second digest

The World Health Organization reports a 'double burden' across the world where 1.9 billion adults are overweight or obese versus the 600 million who are starving. Overweightedness in children is rising 30% faster in developing countries, in line with increasing affluence and adoption of Western dietary patterns. Overweight is defined clinically as a body mass index over 25; obesity is a body mass index over 30. In children, age-related weight for height is used. The physiological causes of obesity are simple: an excess of dietary energy (calories) in relation to energy expended. However, the societal and behavioural drivers are more complex and include cheap, abundant energy-dense foods, marketing and low physical activity levels as a consequence of changes to work, travel, entertainment and domestic life. This means that obesity is difficult to prevent and treat. Obesity impacts adversely on disease risk (especially type 2 diabetes, cancer and cardiovascular disease) and may reduce well-being, increasing risk of depression and lower self-esteem. Efforts to reduce obesity have included population policies, such as limiting the promotion of certain foods or applying sugar taxes, as well as individual actions, such as professional advice, drugs or bariatric surgery.

RELATED TOPICS
See also
FATS
page 22

METABOLISM
page 38

REFINING
page 136

3-SECOND BITE
Despite overweightedness affecting most adults and around a third of children, leading to increased risk of ill health, prevention and treatment strategies have remained largely ineffective.

3-MINUTE SNACK
Obesity has now become the norm in many populations where 24/7 access to affordable, palatable foods is seen as a right, thanks to persuasive advertising. This presents an issue for health legislators, as policies to restrict eating habits and promote physical activity are often viewed as bossy and intrusive. Yet there does remain a hankering after the unattainable thinness of celebrities and the pursuance of faddy diets that don't work in the long term.

3-SECOND BIOGRAPHIES
ADOLPHE QUETELET
1796–1874
Belgian mathematician who devised a way of expressing weight for height in adults: weight (kg) divided by height (m²) – the Body Mass Index.

JOHN GARROW
1929–2006
Scottish-born nutritionist who was one of the first to see the approaching epidemic of obesity and tried to find solutions through meticulous human research.

30-SECOND TEXT
Carrie Ruxton

While the prevalence has begun to slow, no country has managed to reverse obesity.

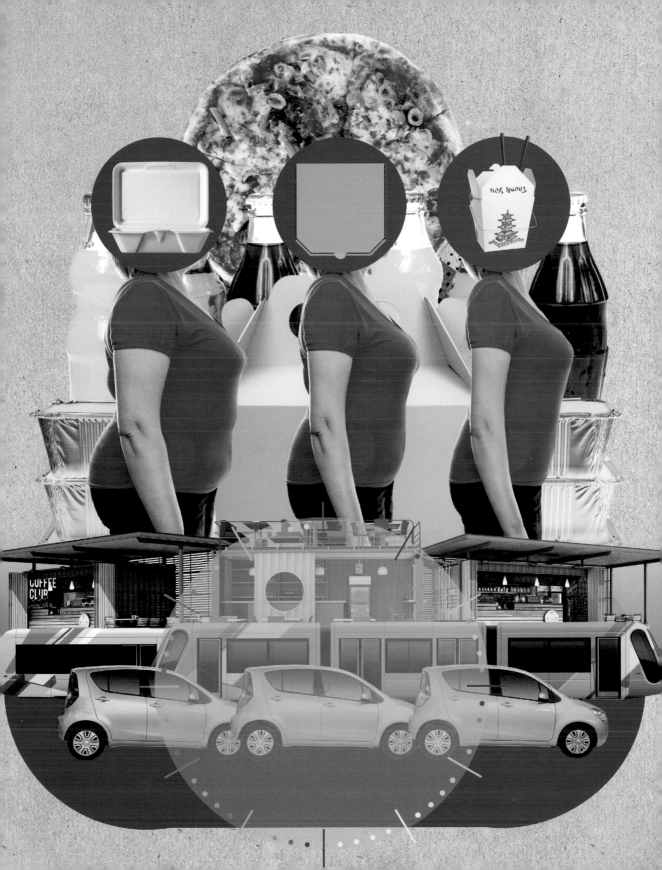

MALNUTRITION

the 30-second digest

Malnutrition occurs when a person doesn't eat enough, through illness, or when there is insufficient amounts or quality of food resulting in insufficient essential nutrients. The consequence is weight loss or reduced growth of children. Symptoms include a lack of interest in eating and drinking, chronic fatigue and a diminished immune system that increases the likelihood of illness and slows recovery. Stunted childhood growth is the most common outcome, resulting from multiple nutritional deficiencies, especially protein, zinc, iodine and milk, which each influence height growth, and an insanitary environment, with a lack of clean water and soap. Kwashiorkor – severe malnutrition with oedema and often with fatty liver and skin changes – most likely reflects tissue and organ damage caused by infections, or dietary toxins and a lack of protective micronutrients, minerals and essential fatty acids. It is often fatal without careful management, which involves antibiotics and cautious feeding with a low-protein feed, electrolytes and multivitamins. Public health programmes focus on clean water and micronutrient supplementation. Obesity is a type of malnutrition in which overconsumption of energy-rich sugary or fatty foods accompany an inactive lifestyle.

RELATED TOPICS
See also
DIETARY ASSESSMENT
page 48

BABIES, INFANTS & CHILDREN
page 76

OVERWEIGHT & OBESITY
page 86

3-SECOND BIOGRAPHIES
JOHN WATERLOW
1916–2010
British scientist who identified fatty liver disease in the Caribbean and Africa, and became a respected authority on childhood malnutrition.

ANN ASHWORTH
1939–
British nutritionist largely responsible for the management regime for severely malnourished children and WHO's '10 steps' approach for inpatient treatment.

30-SECOND TEXT
D Joe Millward

3-SECOND BITE
Malnutrition usually implies inadequate amounts and poor quality food, resulting in weight loss or poor childhood growth, but it can include the wrong sort of food, resulting in obesity.

3-MINUTE SNACK
Malnutrition in adults is identified by weight loss, starting with a body mass index of under 18.5 kg/m², which is associated with increased risk of morbidity and mortality. This could result from illness, so it is common in hospital patients. For children, growth failure or weight loss is assessed as a low weight for age, either through a low weight for height (wasting) or a low height for age (stunting). The latter condition is the most prevalent, with about 25% of pre-school children stunted globally.

The Malnutrition Task Force works to prevent and treat malnutrition in the developing world.

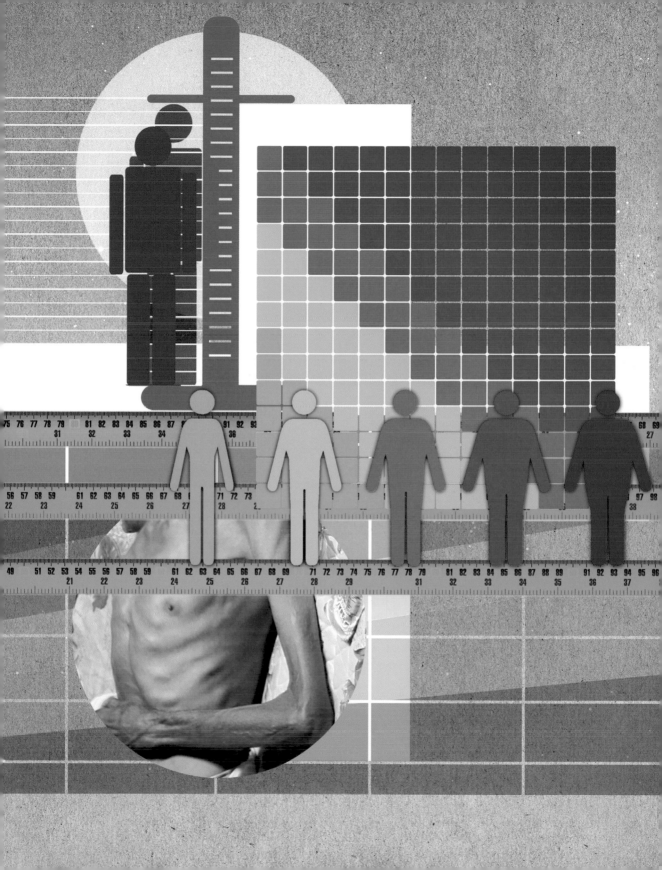

23 September 1880
Born in Kilmaurs,
Scotland, UK

1902–12
Gains degrees in Arts
(1902), Biological Science
(1910) and Medicine (1912)
from Glasgow University

1914
Appointed first Director
of Nutrition Research
Institute in Aberdeen

1914–18
Serves as a medical
officer at the battles
of Somme, Ypres and
Passchendaele, where he
also improves the troops'
diet with local vegetables

1919
Returns to the Institute,
which is renamed the
Rowett Research Institute
in 1922

1932
Elected Fellow of the
Royal Society for his
research on animal and
human nutrition and
agriculture

1940
Appointed an architect
of national wartime food
policy development by
Winston Churchill

1941
Elected first President of
UK Nutrition Society

1945
Appointed as the first
Director General of the
United Nations' Food and
Agriculture Organization

1948
Made Baron of Brechin

1949
Awarded the Nobel
Peace Prize

1968
Made Companion
of Honour

25 June 1971
Dies in Edzell, Scotland

JOHN BOYD ORR

Nobel Laureate Baron John Boyd

Orr, described by some as the 'Scotsman of the twentieth century', was a prodigiously gifted scientist, administrator, champion of the poor and spellbinding broadcaster.

From a religious upbringing in Scotland, Orr won a rare bursary to Kilmarnock Academy, and went on to teach, learn book-keeping and accountancy, and study and practise medicine, before accepting a pivotal two-year research scholarship, which included work on malnutrition and the energy expenditure of military recruits in training. During World War 1, Orr developed his interest in military nutritional and medical welfare, serving with the Infantry and Navy. On return from the War, Orr consolidated his work on the founding of the Rowett Research Institute.

Orr's research was almost certainly responsible for the improved iodine status of the UK population through his recognition of its need in dairy cattle feed, which resulted in its presence in milk, which was eventually provided free or subsidized to school children after the Milk Marketing Board was established in 1933. Because of his writing and broadcasting on the need for a national food policy, given that a third of the population were too poor to buy sufficient food, he became involved with the considerations of the League of Nations for a World Food Plan based on human needs and its publication of the first set of Human Nutritional Requirements.

During World War II, Orr advocated a wartime diet based on government subsidies for essential foods, which eventually became government rationing policy for certain foods, including bacon, butter and sugar, but not others such as bread, potatoes, vegetables, fruit and fish; the use of 85% rather than 70% extraction flour in bread making; and the eventual provision of free cod liver oil, milk and orange juice to all pre-school children.

These wartime policies resulted in a US prize to the British Ministries of Food and Health, which named Boyd Orr amongst those involved. When the United Nations' Food and Agriculture Organization (FAO) was formed in 1945, Orr was invited to be its first Director General, even though he had just been elected as an MP and rector of Glasgow University. He took the post for two years and, although unsuccessful in organizing the means for FAO to eliminate hunger and malnutrition, he did set in place a strong international organization. He retired from FAO in 1948, to assume the role of Chancellor of the University of Glasgow, to write and to travel the world lecturing about food, agriculture, world unity and peace.

D Joe Millward

CHANGING
EATING HABITS

the 30-second digest

As far as healthy food choices

are concerned, we largely know the drill: eat
more fish, fruit and vegetables, and less highly
refined and processed foods. However, eating
habits are considered to play a key part in our
food choices. The term 'habit' can be defined as
an automatic behaviour, learned and repeated
over and over again. If you instinctively grab a
banana to eat first thing each morning in the
kitchen, you have a habit. So, how can we form
new healthy eating habits? Research tells us
that it's a three-step process. Firstly, there is
deliberate *repetition* of the new behaviour.
Then there is a *cue* to trigger practising the new
behaviour. A cue can include recurring places,
times or people. Lastly, there is *rewarding* of
the new eating behaviour. An example of this
three-step process might be: 1. A commitment
to begin eating porridge every morning
(*repetition*); 2. Leaving your bowl and spoon out
in the kitchen the night before (*cue*); 3. Noting
down the energy and alertness that comes
from eating porridge in the morning (*reward*).
Applying this three-step process increases the
likelihood that the new behaviour will become a
healthy eating habit. The new eating behaviour
also needs to be planned, relevant to an
individual's personal circumstances and easy to
perform, so that it can be practised repeatedly.

3-SECOND BITE
Developing new healthy
eating habits begins with
an effortful new eating
behaviour and gradually
becomes effortless and
automatic over time.

3-MINUTE SNACK
Questions remain about
the time it takes for people
to take up and form new
eating habits. Research
shows that between 18 and
254 days is the most likely
time for people to form a
new habit. This variation
depends on the person, the
behaviour and the given
situation. How long it
takes to form eating habits,
therefore, appears to be an
individual matter.

RELATED TOPICS
See also
PERSONALIZED VERSUS
PUBLIC HEALTH ADVICE
page 46

DIETARY ASSESSMENT
page 48

3-SECOND BIOGRAPHIES
WILLIAM JAMES
1842–1910
American philosopher and
psychologist who is credited
with influencing current ideas
of habit in neuroscience.

ANTHONY DICKINSON
1939–
British neuroscientist who has
increased our understanding
of the difference between
habitual and goal-directed
behaviour.

30-SECOND TEXT
Brian Power

*Changing eating habits
takes time; persistence
is key, as is focusing on
the bigger picture of
overall health.*

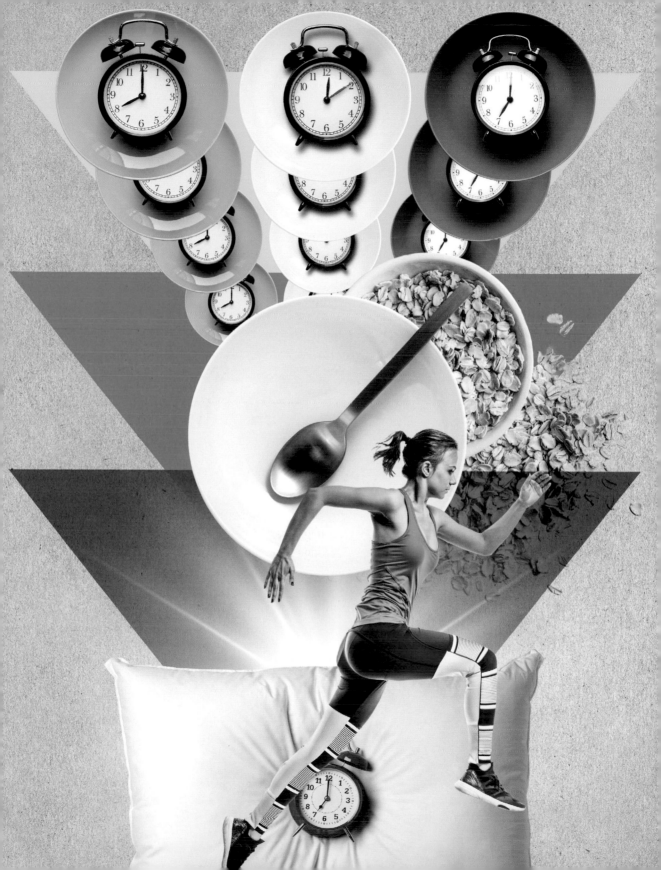

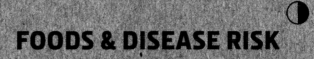

FOODS & DISEASE RISK

acetaldehyde Toxic waste product of alcohol that is a contributing cause of a hangover following alcohol consumption.

anaphylaxis (anaphylactic shock) Severe and potentially life-threatening allergic reaction (see **food allergies**).

blood cholesterol Amount of cholesterol transported in the blood by different lipoproteins. Low density lipoprotein cholesterol (LDL-C) is known as 'bad cholesterol' because it can contribute to the blockage of arteries.

cardiovascular epidemiology The study of how often diseases of the cardiovascular system occur in populations and why.

coeliac disease Specialized food allergy involving an immune response to gluten (found in wheat, barley, rye). The body's response damages the small intestine, causing gastrointestinal symptoms and malabsorption of nutrients.

congeners Substances other than **ethanol** produced during fermentation. Responsible for some of the taste, aroma and colour of alcoholic drinks. Associated with contributing to hangovers; the greatest amounts of these toxins are found in red wine and dark liquors.

coronary heart disease (CHD) When the heart's blood supply is blocked or interrupted by a build-up of fatty substances in the coronary arteries. Symptoms include angina and heart attack.

coronary thrombosis Formation of a blood clot inside a blood vessel of the heart, which restricts blood flow. One of the causes of a heart attack.

ethanol The bulk of ethanol in the body is broken down in the liver by an enzyme called 'alcohol dehydrogenase'.

food allergies Involve an immune response to food and can be severe (**anaphylaxis**) and sometimes fatal. Common foods causing allergy include cows' milk, hens' eggs, fish, shellfish, nuts, peanuts, wheat and soy. Symptoms can include vomiting, diarrhoea, rashes, breathing problems, faintness and loss of consciousness.

food intolerances Disorders of digestion; an inability to break down or take up the food in the normal way. Occur as a response to common foods and are not life-threatening.

fructose Fruit sugar; a simple sugar naturally occurring in fruit, honey, sucrose and high-fructose corn syrup. Very sweet.

glucose A simple one-unit sugar, which is an important source of energy used by the body. 'Blood sugar' refers to the amount of glucose in the blood.

hypertensive Having high blood pressure; rarely has noticeable symptoms. If untreated, it increases risk of serious problems such as heart attacks and strokes.

lactose Sugar found in milk. Broken down into two parts by an enzyme called 'lactase'.

maltose Made out of two glucose molecules bound together, it's created in seeds and other parts of plants. Cereals, certain fruits and sweet potatoes contain high amounts.

monounsaturated fat Dietary fats in which the constituent hydrocarbon chain consists of one carbon–carbon double bond. Often referred to as 'good fats', along with **polyunsaturated fats**, because when substituted for dietary saturated fats they can help lower LDL-cholesterol. Found in avocados, olives, rapeseed oil and some nuts.

normotensive Having normal blood pressure.

phenylketonuria Results from the inability to break down the amino acid phenylalanine (found in many dietary protein sources).

polyphenols Abundant micronutrients found in fruits, vegetables and nuts; evidence for their role in the prevention of degenerative diseases such as cancer and cardiovascular diseases is emerging.

polyunsaturated fat Dietary fats in which the constituent hydrocarbon chain consists of two or more carbon-carbon double bonds. Referred to as 'good fats' because they can help lower LDL-cholesterol. Found in nuts, seeds and oily fish.

saturated fat Dietary fats in which the constituent hydrocarbon chain consists of single carbon–carbon bonds. Referred to as 'bad fats' as high intakes are linked to raised LDL-cholesterol and risk of heart disease.

sodium nitrite Common additive to red meat, due to: inhibiting growth of disease-causing micro-organisms; providing taste and colour; and helping to prevent rancidity.

starch Most abundant carbohydrate in the human diet. Starchy foods include bread, pasta, rice, couscous, potatoes, cereals, oats and other grains like rye and barley.

sucrose Most common dietary disaccharide, containing one glucose and one fructose sugar molecule. From sugar cane or beet.

DIETARY FATS & HEART DISEASE

the 30-second digest

3-SECOND BITE
Reduction of dietary
saturated fats can help to
reduce heart disease, with
greater effects if replaced
by unsaturated fats rather
than simple carbohydrates.

3-MINUTE SNACK
In contrast to the effects
of eating less saturated
fats, consuming long-chain
omega-3 polyunsaturated
fats, chiefly from oily
fish, do not lower blood
cholesterol, but are known
as 'heart healthy' fats
because they confer
protection against heart
disease, heart attacks and
strokes. These effects of
long-chain omega-3 fats
have been attributed to a
reduced tendency of the
blood to clot, improved
function of blood vessels
and stabilization of an
irregular heartbeat.

Saturated fats have been
implicated as one of the main dietary
contributors to heart disease. These fats do
not block our arteries directly, but can raise the
concentration of blood cholesterol, which can
form deposits inside arteries called 'plaques'.
The plaques can then become unstable and
rupture, causing blood clot formation and a
heart attack or stroke. For this reason, dietary
guidelines limit the amount of saturated fats we
should eat. However, this recommendation has
been challenged because of a possible lack of
evidence for a direct relationship between
saturated fats and heart disease mortality, and
the complexity of the relationship between
saturated fats and blood cholesterol. When
we eat less saturated fats, the effect on blood
cholesterol and other risk factors often depends
on what the fats are replaced with. This can
be another type of fat (polyunsaturated or
monounsaturated fat) or carbohydrate, which
will lower blood cholesterol and heart disease
risk, with greater benefits from unsaturated
fats. Not all foods that contain saturated fats
have the same effect on blood cholesterol,
including dairy foods. Compared to butter, the
saturated fats in cheese are absorbed in the gut
to a lesser extent, which reduces the relative
potential of cheese to raise blood cholesterol.

RELATED TOPICS
See also
FATS
page 22

MILK & DAIRY
page 58

OMEGA-3 FATTY ACIDS
page 122

3-SECOND BIOGRAPHIES
ANCEL KEYS
1904–2004
Suggested that hard animal
fats were more important in
influencing blood cholesterol
and risk of coronary heart
disease.

HUGH SINCLAIR
1910–90
First protagonist of the idea
that deficiency of long-chain
omega-3 fatty acids from
marine sources were involved
in coronary thrombosis.

30-SECOND TEXT
Bruce A Griffin &
Julie A Lovegrove

*Diets low in saturated
fats are recommended
to lower blood
cholesterol and reduce
heart disease.*

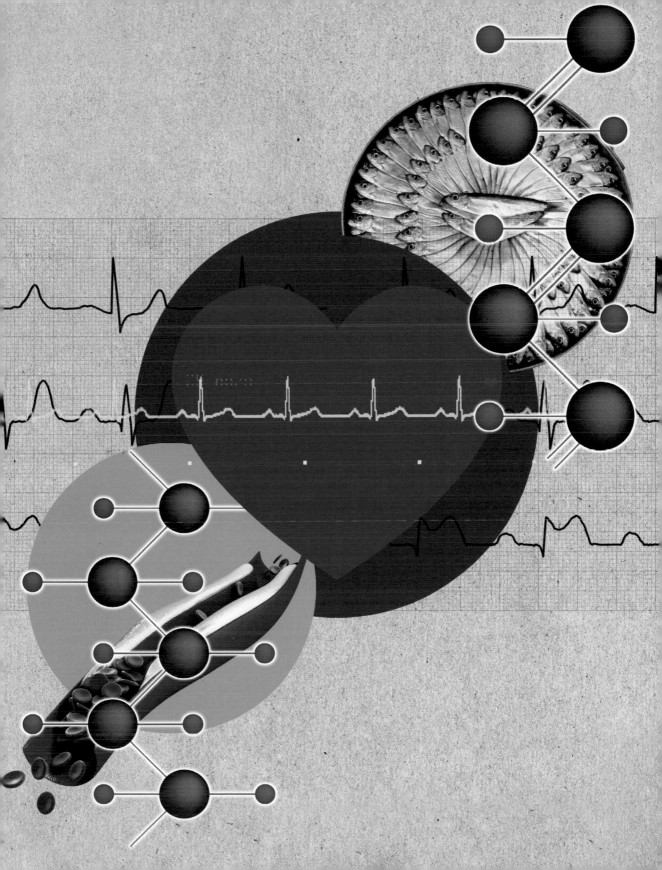

FOOD ALLERGIES & INTOLERANCES

the 30-second digest

Food allergy and intolerance

are adverse reactions to foods, which are dependent on the person rather than the food. Food allergies involve an immune response to food and can be severe (anaphylaxis) and sometimes fatal. Common foods causing allergy include cows' milk, hens' eggs, fish, shellfish, nuts, peanuts, wheat and soy. After consuming the food, symptoms can develop rapidly or be delayed, and include vomiting, diarrhoea, rashes, breathing problems, faintness and loss of consciousness. Coeliac disease is a specialized food allergy involving an immune response to gluten (found in wheat, barley and rye). The body's response damages the small intestine, causing gastrointestinal symptoms and malabsorption of nutrients. Food intolerances are disorders of digestion because of an inability to break down or take up the food in the normal way. They occur as a response to common foods and are not life-threatening. Lactose intolerance results from the reduced ability to break down milk sugar. Commonly screened for at birth, phenylketonuria is the result of an inability to break down the amino acid phenylalanine (found in many dietary protein sources). Management of adverse reactions to food usually requires a physician/dietitian-guided reduction or avoidance of the food.

RELATED TOPICS
See also
NUTS
page 62

GRAINS & GLUTEN
page 64

LABELS & PACKAGING
page 140

3-SECOND BIOGRAPHIES
CHARLES ROBERT RICHET
1850–1935
Awarded the Nobel Prize in Medicine 1913 in recognition of his work on anaphylaxis or 'anti-protection'.

SIR PETER BRIAN MEDAWAR
1950–87
Jointly awarded the Nobel Prize in Medicine in 1960 with Sir Frank Macfarlane Burnet for the discovery of acquired immunological tolerance.

30-SECOND TEXT
Philip C Calder
& Elizabeth A Miles

Reduced intake may be the best management for intolerance; lifelong avoidance is often necessary for allergies.

3-SECOND BITE
Food allergy and food intolerance differ because intolerance does not involve the immune system, whereas allergy is immune-mediated and potentially life-threatening.

3-MINUTE SNACK
The immune system protects against harmful agents but must ignore non-harmful agents or substances (such as food, non-harmful organisms). When the immune system recognizes foods, a tolerant response must be generated to avoid causing unnecessary damage. Food allergy is not so much the appearance of an immune response to a food, but rather the lack of either the generation or maintenance of immune tolerance.

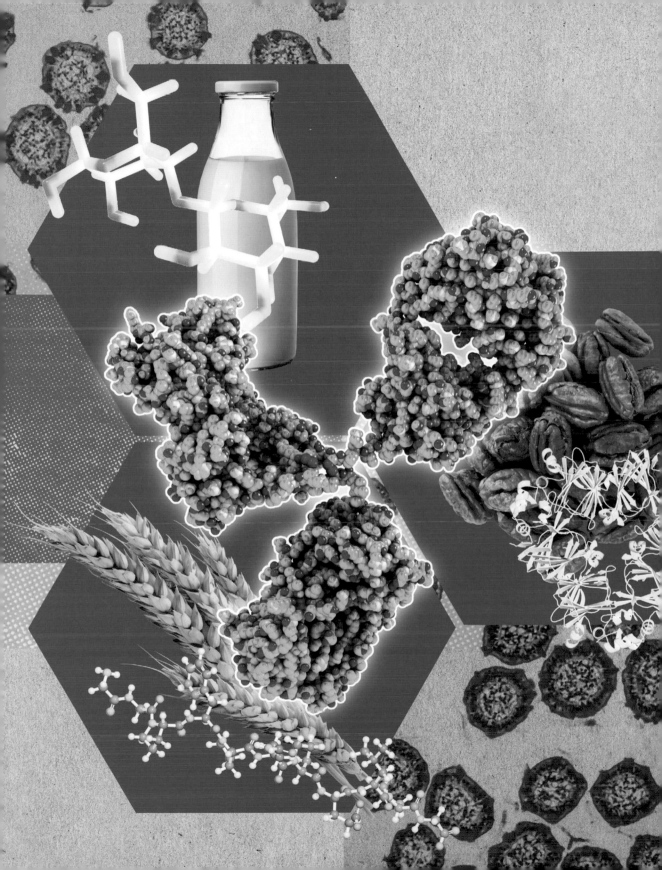

8 August 1910
Born in London, UK

1929
Gains a degree from Chelsea Polytechnic

1931
Graduates with a degree in Physiology and Biochemistry from Christ's College, Cambridge

1933
Marries Milly Himmelweit, a recent emigre from Berlin, with whom he has three sons

1935
Completes a PhD in Microbiology at the Department of Biochemistry, Cambridge

1934–38
While studying for his PhD, qualifies as a medical doctor and begins research at the Dunn Nutritional Laboratory, Cambridge

1939–45
Serves in the Medical Corps and is posted to Sierra Leone where he researches riboflavin (vitamin B2) deficiency in soldiers

1945–54
Becomes Chair of Physiology at Queen Elizabeth College in London, where he develops the first BSc and MSc degrees in Nutrition

1954–71
Elevated to Emeritus Professor of Nutrition at Queen Elizabeth College

1993
Awarded an honorary fellowship of the Hebrew University, Jerusalem

12 July 1995
Dies in London, just four months after the loss of his wife

JOHN YUDKIN

The fact that a 1970s' book on sugar, entitled *Pure, White and Deadly*, still resonates today is testament to the huge impact that Professor John Yudkin had on the theory and practice of nutrition.

Born in the East End of London to Orthodox Russian Jewish parents, Yudkin and his four brothers had a difficult upbringing marked by poverty. Education was a way out, and the young Yudkin quickly discovered how to use his impressive intellect to climb the academic ladder, first at Chelsea Polytechnic in London and later at Cambridge University.

A PhD and medical degree followed in the mid-to-late 1930s. At that time, one had to qualify as a medical doctor in order to become a nutritionist, as there were no specific nutrition courses. This was to change under Yudkin's leadership, when he took up his Chair at Queen Elizabeth College, London.

First, war intervened and took Yudkin to Sierre Leone in West Africa, where he served in the Medical Core as a pathologist. On seeing many soldiers with skin conditions, he discovered that the cause was a deficiency of riboflavin (vitamin B2), not infection as previously believed. Returning from World War II, Yudkin developed his research interests in a number of directions, including enzymes, public health nutrition, diseases of affluence, food choice and historical aspects of diet.

By the mid-1950s, Yukin's concerns switched to obesity, which was at the start of its upward trajectory, and specifically the negative effects of sugar (sucrose). It was Yudkin's view, based on analysis of population diets and disease statistics, that rising intakes of sugar and processed foods were driving the higher rates of obesity, dental decay and chronic diseases seen in wealthier countries. This opinion was consolidated by his success in reducing patients' weight using low carbohydrate diets.

As expert opinion at that time blamed high intakes of dietary fat for cardiovascular diseases, Yudkin often swam against the tide. However, his popular books, *This Slimming Business* and *Pure, White and Deadly*, first published in 1972, resonated with the public, and are still read widely today.

Although Yudkin's research into sugar was later criticized for failing to account for confounding variables, such as smoking and poverty, the central theme – that lower intakes of carbohydrates and sugars could alleviate the risk of obesity and chronic disease – has been vindicated in several contemporary, randomized, controlled trials. For his brave stance, and for championing the embryonic nutrition profession, Professor John Yudkin deserves our recognition.

Carrie Ruxton

SALT &
BLOOD PRESSURE

the 30-second digest

Once considered more valuable
than gold, salt has become a ubiquitous food
ingredient, much maligned by the health
establishment yet eaten daily by millions of
people across the world. Common salt (sodium
chloride) is obtained by evaporating brine, either
in pressure vessels or in salt beds – a traditional
method mostly seen in hot, dry countries. In
ancient times, salt was highly valued and even
used as a form of currency. Now it is produced
on industrial levels, mainly in China and the US.
Salt is used not just to flavour foods but also
to preserve perishable goods such as meat, fish
and vegetables. This was one of the earliest
food safety methods and is still used widely
today. Excess salt intake has been associated
with stomach cancer and raised blood pressure,
a risk factor for heart disease and stroke.
Controlled trials suggest that a fall in salt intake
to 5–6 grammes daily (typical intakes are around
8 grammes) significantly lowers systolic blood
pressure. However, lower sodium intakes do
not consistently translate into reduced mortality
or cardiovascular problems. Black, Asian and
hypertensive people seem to benefit more from
salt reduction than white normotensive people,
in terms of blood pressure. It may be that
some people are genetically responsive to salt
reduction, while others are not.

3-SECOND BITE
Salt intakes remain higher
than recommendations,
but while salt reduction
lowers blood pressure,
there is a lack of evidence
that health improvements
follow for all.

3-MINUTE SNACK
Governments unanimously
recommend wholesale salt
reduction, as we only need
around 1 gram daily for
health. However, clear
evidence that everyone
would benefit is lacking,
and there is a worrying
trend towards higher
cholesterol and
triacylglycerol levels on
lower salt diets. More
consistent effects have
been seen for interventions
such as the Dietary
Approaches to Stop
Hypertension (DASH) diet,
which combine reduced
salt with healthy foods,
such as fish, nuts and
plant foods.

RELATED TOPICS
See also
COOKING, PROCESSING
& PRESERVING
page 134

LABELS & PACKAGING
page 140

3-SECOND BIOGRAPHY
LEWIS DAHL
1914–75
American physician who used
a rat model to discover that
sodium-induced hypertension
was related to genetics as
well as salt intake, and noted
that hypertension was rarely
seen in populations with low
salt intake.

30-SECOND TEXT
Carrie Ruxton

*It takes around three
weeks for your taste
buds to become
accustomed to reduced
amounts of salt.*

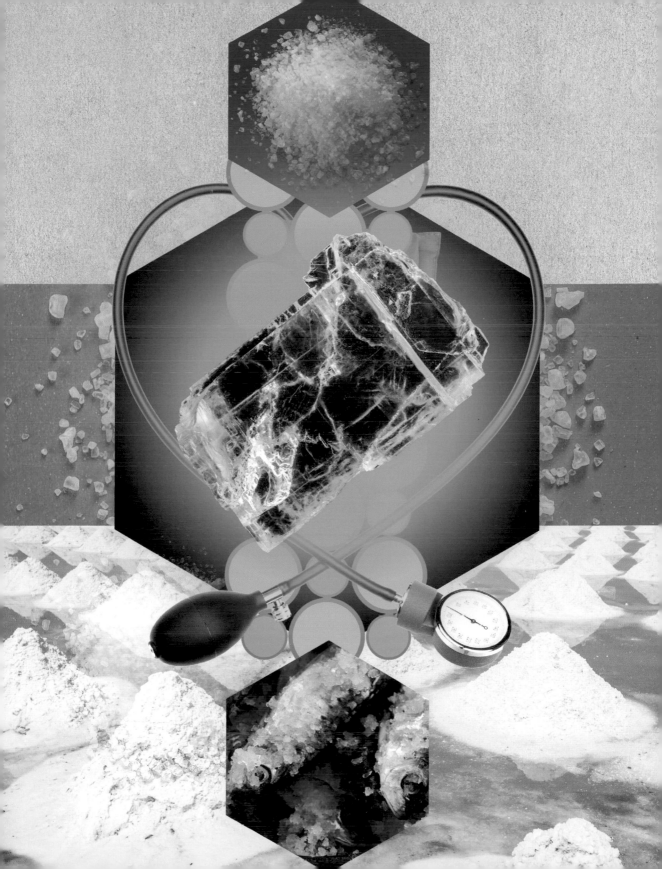

SUGARS & SUGAR SUBSTITUTES

the 30-second digest

3-SECOND BITE
Non-nutritive sweeteners and bulk sugar substitutes could be of benefit in reducing the intake of sugars and the risk of tooth decay and energy overconsumption.

3-MINUTE SNACK
Sugars intake should be reduced to decrease the risk of tooth decay and cavities and of passive overconsumption of energy. The sweetness provided by sugars could be replaced by low-calorie sweeteners, but there are some concerns that this might perpetuate a desire for sweet foods and lead to continued excessive energy intakes. Concerns have been expressed about the safety of sweeteners, but expert reports and research do not support the concerns.

Sweet foods and drinks are perceived as pleasant and highly desirable by the majority of people. In evolutionary terms, this preference was a survival benefit, as it enabled carbohydrate-rich foods, such as fruit, to be identified and consumed, providing a metabolic substrate for the brain. Unfortunately, the desirability of sweet foods can lead to overconsumption of sugars (glucose, fructose, sucrose, maltose) in food and drinks, which in turn can increase the risk of tooth decay, unintentional overconsumption of energy and weight gain. While carbohydrate intake is an essential component of the diet, there is no dietary requirement for sugars, as all of the glucose needed by the brain and other tissues can come from starch. Reducing the sucrose or high-fructose corn syrup content of the diet is challenging if sweet foods and drinks, or products such as cakes and biscuits (in which sucrose has a functional role), are consumed, and so sugar substitutes have to be considered. The replacement of sweetness can be achieved with non-nutritive sweeteners, and reports have shown the safety of these compounds. Replacing the bulk function has not yet been achieved satisfactorily.

RELATED TOPICS
See also
CARBOHYDRATES
page 18

OVERWEIGHT & OBESITY
page 86

REFINING
page 136

3-SECOND BIOGRAPHY
CONSTANTIN FAHLBERG
1850–1910
German–American chemist who discovered the first sweetener, saccharin, after accidentally tasting on his hands a food preservative compound he had just synthesized.

30-SECOND TEXT
Ian Macdonald

The removal from the diet of unnecessary sugars found in sweet foods clearly presents a challenge.

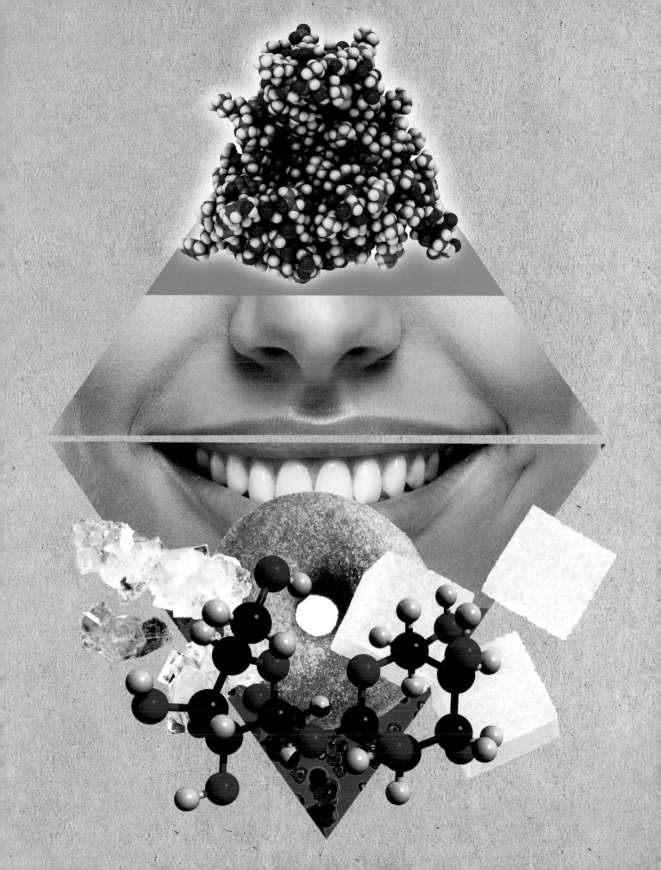

ALCOHOL

the 30-second digest

Whether or not to drink alcohol, especially for 'health purposes', needs careful balancing of the potential benefits with the potential harms. It appears that the difference in health effects lies largely in the dose and patterns of drinking – how much you drink matters more than what you drink. Drinking alcohol in moderation (half a standard glass of wine a day) can generally be beneficial for long-term heart health. On the other hand, when it comes to cancer risk, generally the more alcohol consumed, the higher the long-term risk (particularly breast cancer in women). Whether it's a sip of spirits, wine, liquor or beer, alcohol's active ingredient is the same: ethanol. Alcohol contains other substances, such as polyphenols and congeners, but it's the dose of ethanol that plays the most important role in health effects. The bulk of ethanol in the body is broken down in the liver by an enzyme called 'alcohol dehydrogenase'. Excessive alcohol intake can overwhelm the liver and inflict permanent and serious damage, notably liver cirrhosis (scarring) and cancer. This is due in part, to a build-up of toxic waste products such as acetaldehyde, a contributing cause of hangover following alcohol consumption.

3-SECOND BITE
Drinking no more than 14 units a week spread out over at least three days and with meals may strike the right cancer/heart disease balance in men and women.

3-MINUTE SNACK
Selling alcohol at a minimum price or above it, also known as 'minimum unit alcohol pricing', may produce a variety of health and safety benefits. The basic idea is that minimum unit alcohol pricing can reduce heavy drinking and the associated heart health and cancer problems. This can be achieved by supermarkets targeting cheap, high-strength tipple consumed by the highest-risk drinkers.

RELATED TOPICS
See also
PERSONALIZED VERSUS
PUBLIC HEALTH ADVICE
page 46

DIETARY FATS &
HEART DISEASE
page 98

3-SECOND BIOGRAPHIES
RHAZES
864–930 CE
Pioneering doctor, author and philosopher from Iran; the first to adopt the use of alcohol for medical purposes.

SERGE RENAUD
1927–2012
French researcher who studied the role of alcohol in coronary heart disease; close connection to the French Paradox theory.

30-SECOND TEXT
Brian Power

Fermentation causes the chemical and sensory properties of wine to change, with preservations of aroma and flavour.

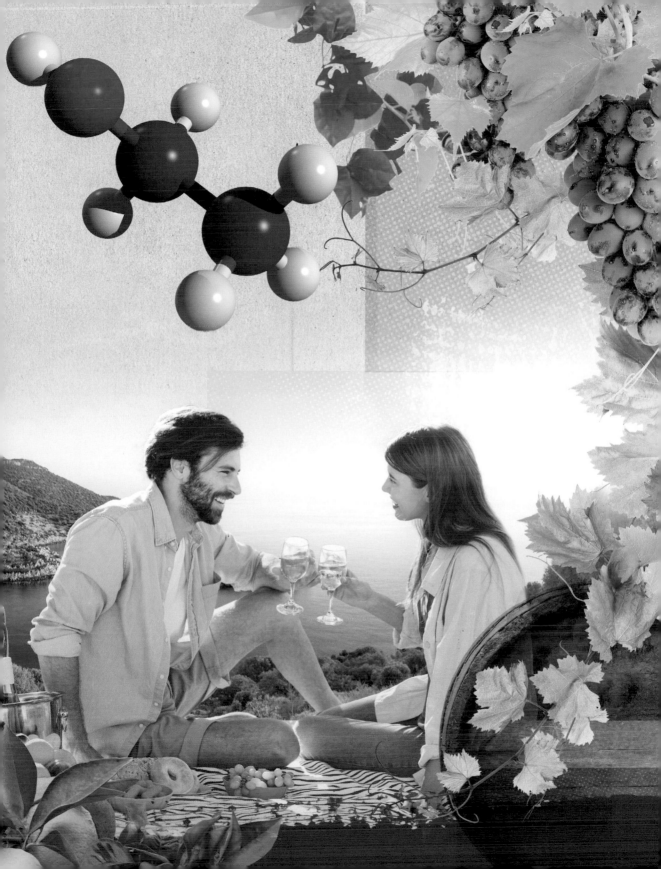

RED & PROCESSED MEAT

the 30-second digest

3-SECOND BITE
Whilst red meat can be nutritious, it should be consumed in moderation; a diet with little processed meat is even more important.

3-MINUTE SNACK
Processing of meat has a long history, with evidence of salting and sun-drying in Ancient Egypt and preservation using snow and ice by early Romans. Nowadays processing is usually to preserve the meat or change its taste by methods including salting, fermentation, smoking or the addition of sodium nitrite.

Red meat includes beef, lamb, pork and venison, and is usually a good source of important nutrients such as high-quality protein, iron, zinc and a number of B vitamins. It is, however, very variable, notably in fat content, which will depend on, for example, the source of the meat, the particular cut and the age of the animal. Processed meat is an even more variable commodity as it is meat that has been transformed through a wide range of processes, and includes sausages, ham, bacon and corned beef. Most processed meat contains beef or pork but can include other meats. There has been much publicity suggesting that consumption of red and processed meat can increase the risk of coronary heart disease, type 2 diabetes and cancer of the large intestine and rectum. The hard evidence is clear: the risk of these diseases from the consumption of processed meat is substantially greater than from red meat. For example, the risk of intestinal cancer from processed meat is about twice of that from red meat. It is, therefore, important to maintain a low consumption of processed meat.

RELATED TOPICS
See also
DIETARY FATS & HEART DISEASE
page 98

NITRATE & NITRITE
page 118

FREE-RANGE & INTENSIVELY FARMED FOODS
page 144

3-SECOND BIOGRAPHIES
NICOLAS APPERT
1749–1841
French inventor of airtight food preservation who has been described as the 'father of canning'.

CLARENCE BIRDSEYE II
1886–1956
American inventor regarded as the founder of food preservation by freezing, especially fast freezing.

30-SECOND TEXT
Ian Givens

WHO now labels processed meats as 'carcinogenic to humans' and red meat as 'probably carcinogenic'.

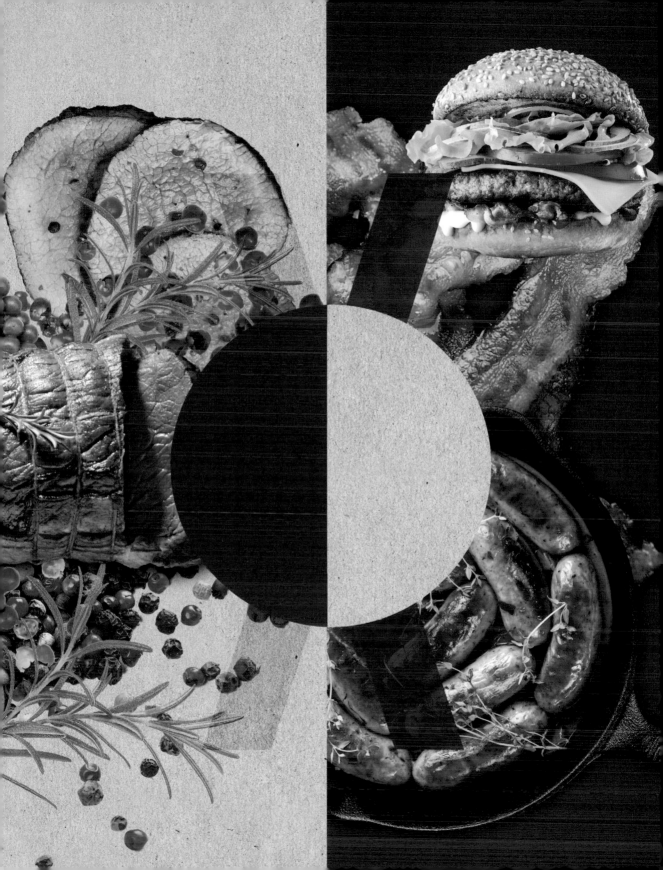

POTENTIAL BIOACTIVES & HEALTH

POTENTIAL BIOACTIVES & HEALTH
GLOSSARY

alpha-linolenic acid Essential **fatty acid** found in nuts and seeds; a metabolic precursor of long chain omega-3 fatty acids, particularly eicosapentaenoic acid (EPA) and docosahexaenoic acid (DHA).

Alzheimer's disease See **dementia**.

amines Derivatives of ammonia; released by the breakdown of amino acids. Many neurotransmitters are amines, including dopamine, serotonin and histamine. Can be found in cheese, wine and chocolate.

atherosclerosis Build-up of material, including cholesterol, inside arteries; causes narrowing of the arteries, which, when blocked by a blood clot (thrombus), causes heart attacks and strokes.

bifidobacteria Major type of bacteria that make up the gut microbiome. Some are used as probiotics. Found in foods such as live-culture yoghurt.

dementia Syndrome associated with an ongoing decline of brain functioning. Affects memory, thinking speed, language, understanding, judgement, mood and movement. Alzheimer's disease is the most common cause.

fatty acids (FAs) The building blocks of fat in the body and in food. During digestion, the body breaks down fats into FAs, which can then be absorbed into the blood.

flavonoids Common chemical compounds that are present in many plant-based foods and drinks, such as blueberries, tea, citrus fruits, wine, onions and chocolate.

glucosinolates Main phytochemical found in cruciferous crops. Epidemiological and experimental data suggests they may act as anti-carcinogenic agents.

hypertension High blood pressure; rarely has noticeable symptoms. If untreated, it increases risk of heart attacks and strokes. Can be decreased by reducing salt, cutting back on alcohol, losing weight and exercising.

isoflavones Class of **flavonoids**, which are produced only by members of the bean family of plants (*Fabaceae*).

isothiocyanates Produced by *Brassicales* plants to defend against pests and diseases. When these plants are eaten, an enzyme converts **glucosinolate** molecules in the plant tissues into isothiocyanates, creating distinctive aromas and flavours. May be effective against types of cancer.

lactobacilli 'Friendly' bacteria that live in the digestive, urinary and genital systems without causing disease; associated with beneficial health effects. Also found in some fermented foods like yoghurt and in dietary supplements.

microbiota Billions of bacteria living in the large intestine. The bacteria live in a symbiotic relationship with their human hosts, influencing a wide range of bodily processes – positively and negatively.

neurodegenerative Range of conditions which primarily affect the neurons in the human brain. Diseases include Parkinson's, **Alzheimer's** and Huntington's.

nitric oxide Gas naturally produced in the body; used to communicate between cells; cardio-protective.

osteomalacia Rickets in adults.

osteoporosis Bone-weakening condition that develops over years until a fall or impact causes a bone fracture. Postmenopausal women are at risk.

polyphenols Abundant substances found in fruits, vegetables and nuts; evidence for their role in the prevention of degenerative diseases such as cancer and cardiovascular diseases is emerging. **Flavonoids** and **isoflavones** belong to this compound class.

polyunsaturated fats Dietary fats in which the constituent hydrocarbon chain consists of two or more carbon-carbon double bonds. Referred to as 'good fats' because they can help lower LDL-cholesterol.

prebiotics Indigestible components of food that are able to reach the large intestine, to feed beneficial bacteria and promote its growth and function.

probiotics Micro-organisms claimed to provide health benefits (especially gut-related) when consumed. Added to yoghurts or taken as supplements; 'good' or 'friendly' bacteria.

rickets Children's skeletal disorder leading to softening of the bones; caused by a lack of vitamin D or calcium.

sulforaphane Isothiocyanate found in broccoli and rocket; may be associated with lower risk of prostrate cancer.

type 1 diabetes Failure of the pancreas to produce insulin, which results in glucose remaining in the blood rather than being taken up by cells and used as fuel for energy.

FLAVONOIDS & ISOFLAVONES

the 30-second digest

3-SECOND BITE
Flavonoids and
isoflavones are common
chemical compounds that
are present in many of
the plant-based foods
and drinks we consume
every day.

3-MINUTE SNACK
Flavonoids and
isoflavones belong to a
class of compounds called
'polyphenols'. This group
also contains anthocyanins
(present in grapes and red
wine), catechins (found
in cocoa) and phenolic
acids (found in anything
from artichokes to wine).
These compounds are also
thought to impart health
benefits in humans, though
the exact mechanisms by
which this happens are
not always apparent. Gut
microbial populations may
play an important role.

Flavonoids and isoflavones are compounds produced by plants and fungi, which can act as colour pigments in flowers, a defence against high UV light and as a chemical defence against some plant diseases. Flavonoids are present in many of the fruits and vegetables that we eat and drink, such as blueberries, green and black tea, citrus fruits, wine, onions and cocoa. There is some evidence to suggest that consuming these compounds and their metabolites reduces the risk of developing conditions such as atherosclerosis, reduces blood pressure and improves vascular function. Relatively recent research has shown that specific compounds may reduce cognitive decline, which is linked with improvements in vascular health, increased blood flow and maintaining synaptic connections in the brain. Isoflavones are similar to flavonoids, but are produced only by members of the bean family of plants (*Fabaceae*) – soy, green beans and peanuts. The health benefits of isoflavones are not as well studied as flavonoids, but there are clinical indications that consumption decreases cancer risk in postmenopausal women and reduces some risk factors of cardiovascular disease.

RELATED TOPICS
See also
GUT MICROBIOME
page 40

FRUIT & VEGETABLES
page 54

POSTMENOPAUSAL WOMEN
page 82

3-SECOND BIOGRAPHIES
JUNJI TERAO
1951–
World leader in the metabolic
effects of flavonoids and
isoflavones.

JEREMY SPENCER
1971–
Leading researcher in the
effects of polyphenols
on cognition.

30-SECOND TEXT
Luke Bell

*Isoflavones are present
in processed foods such
as tofu and miso soup
in high concentrations.*

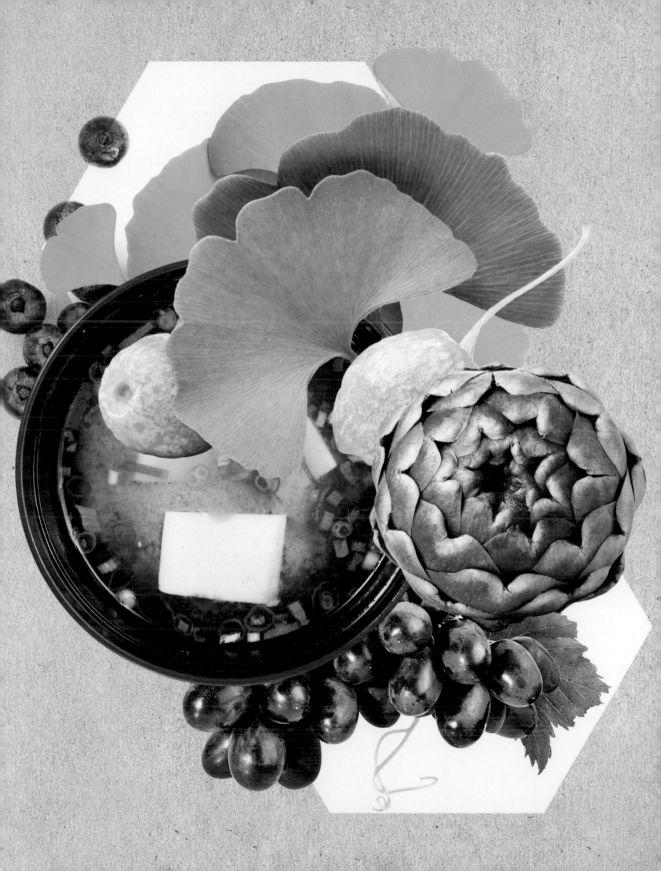

NITRATE & NITRITE

the 30-second digest

Nitrate was previously thought to be an inert end product of body metabolism. However, research over the last decade or so has revealed nitrate and nitrite to be important molecules for production of cardio-protective nitric oxide. Nitrate is found naturally in vegetables, particularly green leafy varieties and beetroot. Studies have shown that the consumption of dietary nitrate dramatically lowers blood pressure as well as improving physical performance. These effects are mediated by the conversion of nitrate to nitrite by bacteria in the mouth, followed by conversion to nitric oxide in blood vessels. This causes the vessels to relax and dilate, increasing blood flow and lowering blood pressure. In contrast, the consumption of nitrate and nitrite in processed meat has been associated with an increased risk of colon cancer. Nitrate and nitrite are often added to processed meat to prevent microbial spoilage and to preserve its red colour. Yet, under the acidic environment of the stomach, nitrite may react with compounds called 'amines', found in meat to produce nitrosamines – known carcinogens. However, vegetables have low levels of amines, and contain vitamin C and polyphenolic compounds that favour the production of nitric oxide and reduce the formation of nitrosamines.

RELATED TOPICS

See also
FRUIT & VEGETABLES
page 54

RED & PROCESSED MEAT
page 110

3-SECOND BIOGRAPHIES
ROBERT F FURCHGOTT &
LOUIS J IGNARRO
1916–2009 & 1941–
American biochemists who discovered the role of nitric oxide as an important signalling molecule in the cardiovascular system.

30-SECOND TEXT
Ditte Hobbs

Beetroot juice has been used to increase performance in elite athletes, as well as helping the body cope with high altitudes.

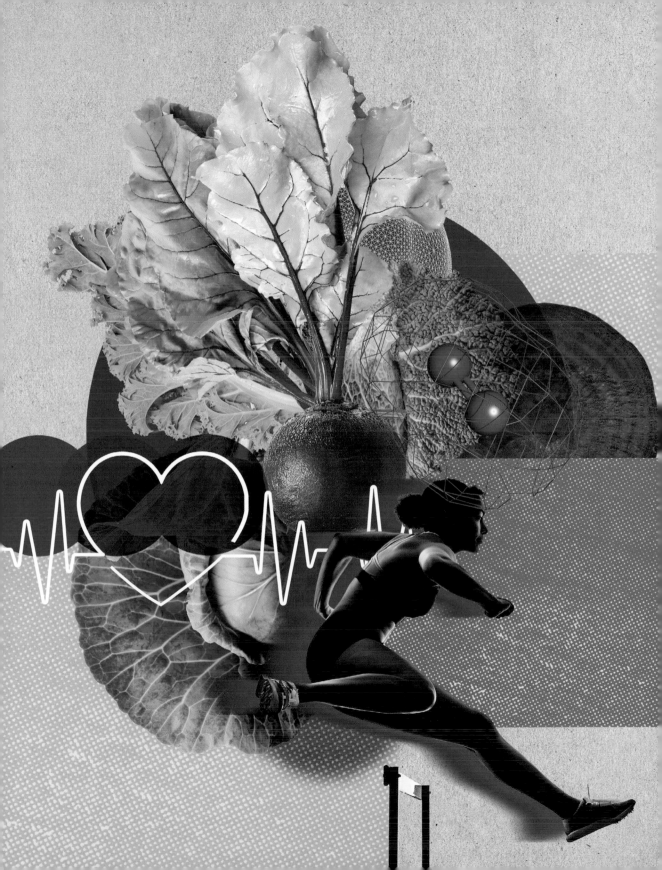

ISOTHIOCYANATES

the 30-second digest

Brassicales plants produce
isothiocyanates to defend themselves
against pests and diseases. They are the
reason why cabbage smells sulfurous, why
mustard is hot and why you may hate the
taste of Brussels sprouts at Christmas. When
these plants are eaten, an enzyme converts
glucosinolate molecules in the plant tissues into
isothiocyanates, creating distinctive aromas
and flavours. Some isothiocyanates also
happen to be effective against types of cancer.
Sulforaphane is an isothiocyanate found in
broccoli and rocket, and can help prevent and
slow the progression of prostate cancer. People
who eat a greater proportion of *Brassica*-type
vegetables in their diets (kale, cabbage, broccoli)
are at a lower risk of developing chronic
diseases such as cancer, heart disease and
neurodegenerative conditions. Cooking by
boiling, steaming or microwaving is very bad
for the enzyme that produces isothiocyanates,
as it breaks down at temperatures above 60°C
(140°F). Stir-frying helps to maintain the health
benefits, and eating raw salads with watercress
and rocket is a good way to include them in the
diet, without the need for cooking.

3-SECOND BITE
Isothiocyanates are
important dietary
components for the
reduction in risk of certain
chronic diseases and are
also responsible for the
flavours of foods such
as mustard and cabbage.

3-MINUTE SNACK
With an ageing population,
diseases such as cancer and
dementia are becoming
more prevalent in society.
Eating vegetables that
contain isothiocyanates
on a regular basis may be
associated with lowering
the risk of developing some
cancers and forms of
neurodegeneration.
Isothiocyanate compounds
interact with our genes and
promote metabolism of
cellular waste products
in a less harmful way,
which protects our DNA
from damage.

RELATED TOPICS
See also
NUTRIENT–GENE
INTERACTIONS
page 42

FRUIT & VEGETABLES
page 54

3-SECOND BIOGRAPHY
RICHARD MITHEN
1960–
British professor who produced
the world's first 'super
broccoli' that has increased
amounts of the isothiocyanate
sulforaphane.

30-SECOND TEXT
Luke Bell

*Research strongly
suggests that we
should develop a
healthy love for
Brassica vegetables.*

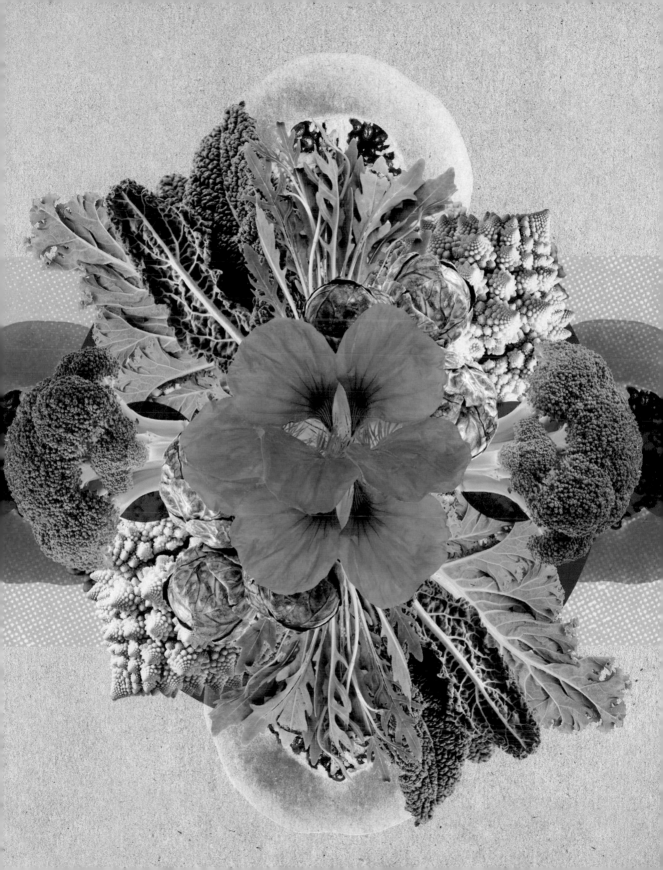

OMEGA-3 FATTY ACIDS

the 30-second digest

3-SECOND BITE
Omega-3 fatty acids are important for maintaining human health. The best source of the most important omega-3 fatty acids (EPA and DHA) is fatty fish.

3-MINUTE SNACK
EPA and DHA change cell membrane structure and function, regulate the chemical signals produced by cells and control the genes that cells express. Through these actions, EPA and DHA modify cell and tissue behaviour and responses in a way that optimizes function, thereby improving health and reducing disease risk. The sustainability of fish as a source of EPA and DHA is not certain.

Omega-3 fatty acids are a class of polyunsaturated fats. They are rarer in most diets than saturated, monounsaturated and omega-6 polyunsaturated fats. Omega-3 fatty acids come from plants and animals. The main plant omega-3 fatty acid is alpha-linolenic acid. This cannot be made in animals and is an essential fatty acid. The main role of alpha-linolenic acid is as a metabolic precursor of more complex omega-3 fatty acids, particularly eicosapentaenoic acid (EPA) and docosahexaenoic acid (DHA). However, this metabolic conversion is relatively inefficient and humans need preformed EPA and DHA to support cell function and to maintain health. The main dietary source of EPA and DHA is seafood, especially fatty fish (salmon, tuna, sardines, mackerel). If people do not eat fatty fish, their intake of EPA and DHA is likely to be lower than recommended (around 200 to 500 mg of EPA plus DHA per day). Getting sufficient EPA and DHA is important for health. DHA has key roles in the structure and function of the eye and brain and getting enough DHA early in life, when these organs are developing, is vital. EPA and DHA are important for heart and cognitive health and for the control of inflammation. EPA and DHA are available in supplements, often referred to as fish oils.

RELATED TOPICS
See also
FATS
page 22

FISH
page 56

DIETARY FATS & HEART DISEASE
page 98

3-SECOND BIOGRAPHIES
HANS OLAF BANG & JORN DYERBERG
Danish researchers who travelled to Greenland in the 1970s and early 1980s to study the diet and disease patterns of the Inuit; demonstrated that the reported cardio protection was most likely due to dietary EPA and DHA.

HUGH SINCLAIR
1910–90
British researcher amongst the first to claim that diseases like heart disease were influenced by dietary fats.

30-SECOND TEXT
Philip C Calder

Fittingly, 'omega' means 'great O' (ō mega, mega meaning 'great').

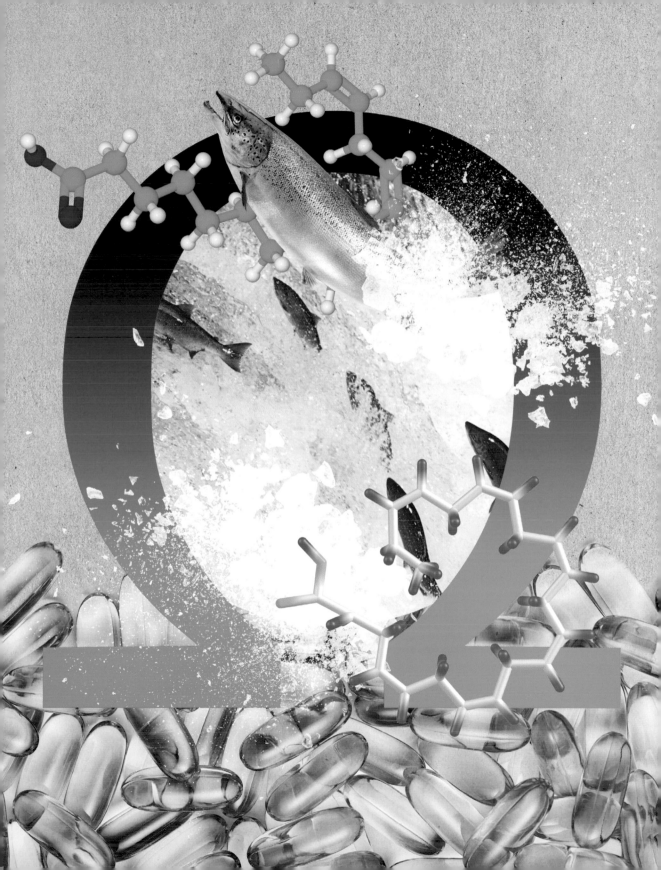

4 February 1910
Born in Edinburgh, UK

1923
Studies at Stone House School then Winchester College, where he is awarded the Headmaster's Natural Science Prize (1928) and the Senior Science Prize (1929)

1933
Awarded the Gotch Memorial Prize

1937
Receives the Radcliffe Travelling Fellowship, which allows Sinclair to make an extensive visit to many of the laboratories in the US and Canada engaged in nutritional research

1942–47
Director of the Oxford Nutrition Survey

1945
Awarded the Chevalier of the Order of Oranje-Nassau by the Queen of the Netherlands for work on the survey of the Dutch population after the Siege of Leningrad

1946
Awarded Honorary Brigadier and, subsequently, the US Presidential Medal of Freedom with Silver Palm, for work on the Oxford Nutrition Survey

1951
Invited to give the Cutter Lecture at Harvard, USA – a prestigious lecture founded in 1912; University Reader in Human Nutrition, Magdalen College, Oxford

1956
Publication of 'Deficiency of essential fatty acids and atherosclerosis, etcetera' in *The Lancet*

1967–68
Master of the Worshipful Society of Apothecaries

1968
Awarded an Honorary DSc from Baldwin-Wallace College

1976
Joins the expedition of Drs Bang and Dyerberg in northwest Greenland, renewing his interest in the Inuit diet

1979
Undergoes his infamous 'Eskimo diet' study

1983–1990
President of the McCarrison Society

22 June 1990
Dies at the age of 80 in Oxford, UK

1995
The Hugh Sinclair Unit of Human Nutrition at the University of Reading is founded, and Sinclair's archive is held in the Museum of English Rural Life (MERL)

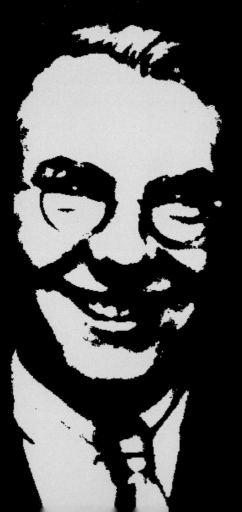

HUGH MACDONALD SINCLAIR

Hugh Macdonald Sinclair was a passionate nutritionist who dedicated his life to investigating diet and chronic disease, and enjoyed an illustrious career in terms of awards and accolades. Nevertheless, his major contributions to the field of human nutrition were not fully recognized in his lifetime by his peers. Sinclair was born in Edinburgh, Scotland, to Rosalie Sybil Jackson and Colonel Hugh Montgomerie Sinclair, a claimed descendent of Woldonius, the Viking monarch of Finland and the St Clair cousins of William the Conqueror.

After attaining a first-class degree in Animal Physiology from Oriel College Oxford and Doctorate of Medicine from University College London, amongst other degrees, he was elected as University Demonstrator and Lecturer in Biochemistry and as a Fellow of Magdalen College Oxford. At the age of 31, the Ministry of Health invited Sinclair to set up the Oxford Nutrition Survey, to establish the health and diet of the British population during World War II. Between 1942 and 1947 Sinclair and his team of 24 staff conducted detailed surveys, not only in the UK but also in Germany and the Netherlands. While this survey was an outstanding achievement, on which the British Government based its rationing strategy, the results were, sadly, never published.

Another landmark achievement in Sinclair's life was recognition of the importance of dietary long-chain omega-3 polyunsaturated fats, found in fish oils, in reducing blood clotting and heart disease risk. This originated from a trip to Greenland to study snow blindness, where Sinclair noticed that the Inuit population did not seem to suffer from heart disease. In 1956 Sinclair published his famous paper, entitled 'Deficiency of essential fatty acids and atherosclerosis, etcetera', in *The Lancet*, a prestigious medical journal, in which he speculated on the links between long-chain omega-3 polyunsaturated fats and heart disease and cancer. Unfortunately, his peers were sceptical, and Sinclair struggled to secure funding for his research to confirm these speculations. This led to his famous 'Eskimo diet' study, when, at the age of 69, he ate nothing but seal meat, fish and water for 100 days, while cutting his arm frequently to measure the time it took for his blood to clot. Remarkably, this diet increased his blood clotting time from 3 to 50 minutes and provided an elegant demonstration of how these fats reduce blood clots in arteries (thrombosis), thereby decreasing risk of a heart attack. This finding was confirmed by other studies, which form the basis for the dietary recommendation to increase intakes of these fats to reduce heart disease.

Julie A Lovegrove

VITAMIN D & CALCIUM

the 30-second digest

Vitamin D is a vitamin in food

that becomes a hormone inside the body. Sunlight supplies most requirements except in northern regions during winter, when dietary sources become important, such as oily fish and eggs. Calcium is a mineral found in dairy foods, green vegetables, nuts and seeds. Vitamin D supports bone health by boosting calcium absorption in the gut and promoting uptake by the bone matrix. Low vitamin D can lead to rickets in children and osteomalacia and osteoporosis in adults. Taking calcium with vitamin D improves bone density and lowers the risk of fractures, particularly in postmenopausal women. There are hundreds of vitamin D receptors in the body, suggesting a wider influence. Studies have reported associations between low vitamin D status (blood levels) and a higher risk of cancer or heart disease. Other research notes that children are at greater risk of type 1 diabetes if their mothers were low in vitamin D during pregnancy. Further evidence is needed to confirm these findings. Vitamin D deficiency is common in western and northern countries, affecting 15 to 40% of the population. Those who are obese or have darker skins are more at risk. Recommendations are 10–20 mg daily, and some countries advise daily supplementation as natural sources are limited.

RELATED TOPICS
See also
BABIES, INFANTS & CHILDREN
page 76

PREGNANCY & LACTATION
page 80

POSTMENOPAUSAL WOMEN
page 82

3-SECOND BIOGRAPHIES
ALFRED HESS
1875–1933
American physician who discovered that cod liver oil and exposure to UV light could cure rickets. He shared in the Nobel prize money awarded to Adolf Windaus for research into rickets.

ELMER MCCOLLUM
1879–1967
American scientist credited with isolating vitamin D and creating the vitamin naming system with Cornelia Kennedy.

30-SECOND TEXT
Carrie Ruxton

The hard framework for bones (cortical) and teeth (enamel) is composed of calcium phosphate.

3-SECOND BITE
Vitamin D deficiency is common in developed countries as year-round sunlight is scarce. Vitamin D works with calcium to maintain bone structure.

3-MINUTE SNACK
Warnings about skin cancer could have inadvertently led to an epidemic in vitamin D deficiency, due to sun avoidance or potentially the use of sun block. Rickets is on the rise, as is osteoporosis. An ideal balance is to get 15 to 20 minutes in the sun daily during summer and to take a supplement in winter.

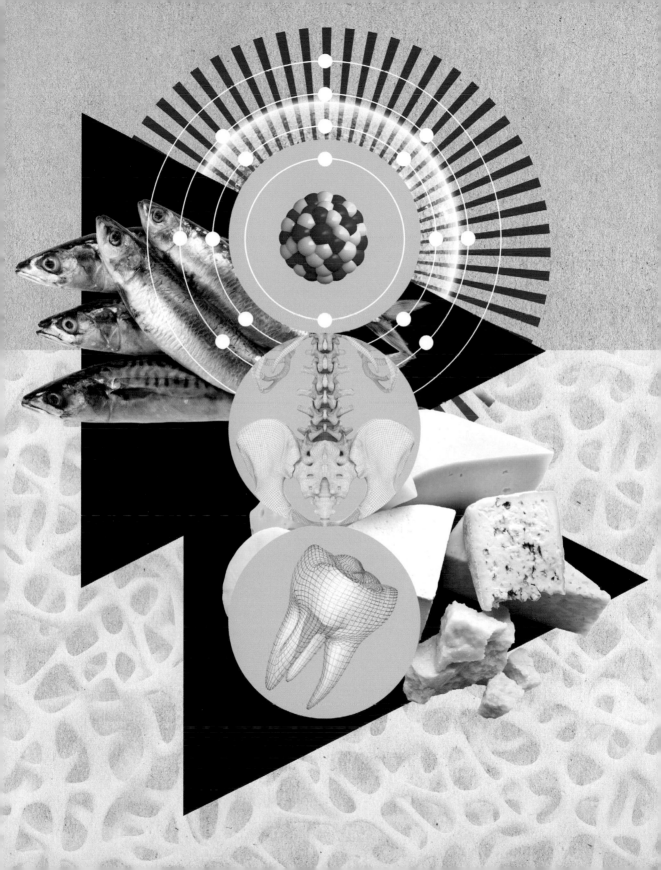

PROBIOTICS & PREBIOTICS

the 30-second digest

Gut health means more than digestive health. The billions of bacteria ('microbiota') in the large intestine live in a symbiotic relationship with their human hosts, influencing a wide range of bodily processes via their proliferation and metabolic activities. In the case of potentially pathogenic bacteria, the impact on health can be negative. However, others such as *bifidobacteria* and *lactobacilli* are associated with beneficial effects such as pathogen inhibition, rebalancing of immune function, blood lipid reduction and metabolic changes that may assist control of weight. Probiotics are live bacteria which, when administered in adequate amounts, confer a health benefit; prebiotic fibres are selectively fermented ingredients, for example inulin-type fructans, galacto-oligosaccharide and lactulose, that change the composition and/or activity of the microbiota to deliver benefits. Do probiotics and prebiotics work? The literature has expanded rapidly and many studies have shown positive outcomes, particularly in relation to infection control, mineral absorption and metabolic effects, some inconsistencies in results are apparent. So, it's a cautious 'yes'.

The large intestine is home to billions of different bacteria, weighing in at 1–2 kg (2.2–4.4 lb).

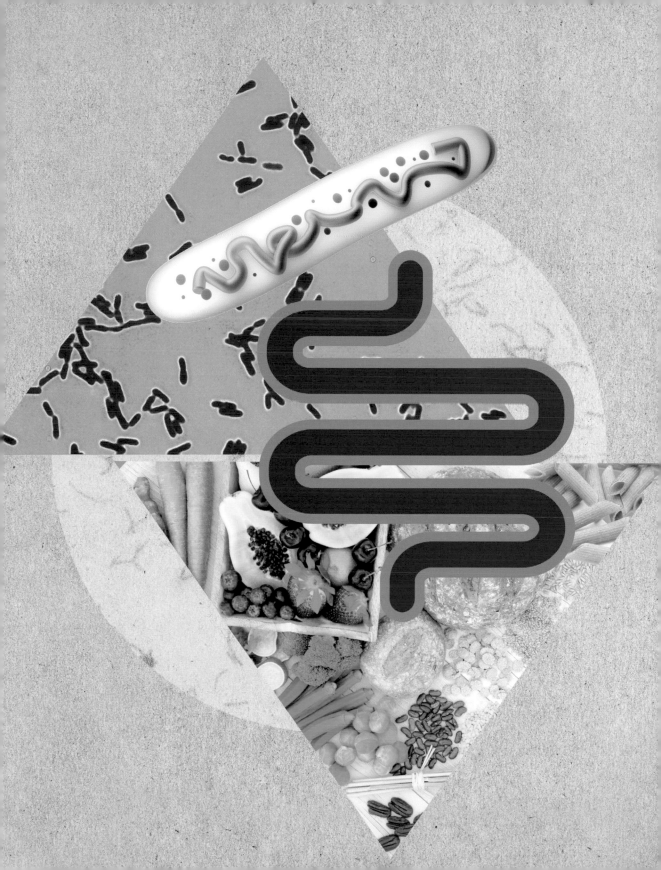

FOOD PROCESSING & PRODUCTION SYSTEMS
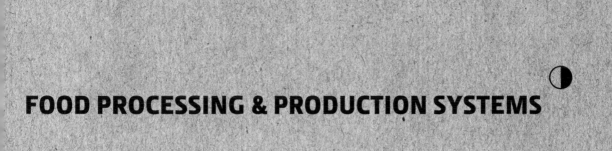

FOOD PROCESSING & PRODUCTION SYSTEMS
GLOSSARY

additives Components added intentionally to a food to affect its characteristic, by improving look or appeal.

ascorbic acid Micronutrient, also known as vitamin C, that also acts as a preservative, antioxidant or colour stabilizer in foods.

beta-lactoglobulin Specific protein in the whey component in milk that can initiate an allergy in some susceptible individuals.

bioavailability Extent to which nutrients are digested and absorbed.

endosperm Food reserve tissue inside the seeds of most flowering plants that surrounds the embryo and provides nutrition in the form of starch. May also contain oils and protein.

enrichment Process that can reintroduce nutrients to **refined foods**, to improve the nutritional quality.

ethical omnivorism Philosophy and diet that makes it essential only to consume foods that come from animals that are grass fed and free range; similarly, only wild fish caught ethically or sustainably farmed fish can be consumed.

gene Basic physical and functional unit of heredity, a specific region of DNA that codes for RNA, which make proteins.

genetic modification or engineering
Genetically modified (GM) organisms are those whose genetic material (DNA) has been altered in a way that doesn't occur naturally through reproduction. Scientists introduce a new gene from a different organism, even one unrelated to the modified species. Has seen the rise of commercialized genetically modified crops and livestock.

iodine Essential micronutrient in the diet, involved in the production of thyroid hormone. Present naturally in soil and seawater; found in dairy products and seafood. Symptoms of deficiency are related to the thyroid.

lycopene Naturally occurring carotenoid that is responsible for the red/pink colours seen in tomatoes, pink grapefruit and other foods.

nitrate Occurs in vegetables, grains and drinking water; produced for use as fertilizers in agriculture. Scientific reviews have reported that organic food crops can contain less nitrate than conventional crops, the consumption of which has been associated with both good and negative effects on health.

polyunsaturated fats Dietary fats in which the constituent hydrocarbon chain consists of two or more carbon–carbon double bonds. Often referred to as 'good fats', along with monounsaturated fats, because when substituted for dietary saturated fats they can help lower LDL cholesterol. Found in nuts, seeds and oily fish.

refined foods Processed or altered foods that are no longer in their natural state, a process that results in a loss of beneficial nutrients and fibre.

saturated fat Dietary fats in which the constituent hydrocarbon chain consists of only single carbon–carbon bonds. Often referred to as 'bad fats' because high intakes are linked to raised LDL-cholesterol and increased risk of heart disease events. Commonly found in animal-derived products.

scurvy Severe vitamin C deficiency. Symptoms include fatigue, weakness, severe joint or leg pain, bleeding gums, red or blue spots on the skin, easy bruising.

selenium Essential mineral that increases immunity, defends against free radical damage and inflammation and maintains a healthy metabolism. Found in Brazil nuts, eggs, liver, tuna, cod, sunflower seeds, poultry and certain types of meat.

World Health Organization (WHO) Agency of the United Nations tasked with building a better, healthier future for people all over the world.

COOKING, PROCESSING & PRESERVING

the 30-second digest

Cooking, processing and preserving have existed since humans began to eat. Cooking makes foods softer, prolongs their life and combines foods to create specific dishes. It is a form of processing and preservation. The application of heat or an acid serves to deactivate naturally occurring enzymes that promote reactions such as browning or ageing, and eventual spoilage. Processing transforms ingredients by physical or chemical means into other forms. It combines raw food ingredients to produce products that are easily prepared and served. There are many methods, including mincing and emulsifying. Preservation prevents the growth of microorganisms such as yeasts, although some methods work by introducing benign bacteria or fungi to the food, as well as slowing the oxidation of fats that cause rancidity. For all three processes, there are pros and cons. Advantages include: less spoilage by prolonging the life of the food; increased availability of the foodstuff and increased bioavailability of some nutrients; reduced food-borne diseases; convenience; enhancing flavour and texture. Disadvantages include: decreased levels of some nutrients (heat destroys vitamin C); use of additives; contamination risks; some methods have been linked to carcinogens; environmental concerns.

RELATED TOPICS
See also
REFINING
page 136

ADDITIVES
page 138

FOOD SUSTAINABILITY
page 148

3-SECOND BIOGRAPHY
NICOLAS APPERT
1749–1841
Looking for ways to feed troops, Napoleon Bonaparte offered a prize for the development of a process to preserve foods. Confectioner and chef Appert rose to the challenge with canning, and the rest is, as they say, history.

30-SECOND TEXT
Judith Rodriguez

3-SECOND BITE
Done properly, cooking provides benefits related to food preservation and nutrient availability, but done improperly, as with overcooking, it may destroy other nutrients and overly process foods.

3-MINUTE SNACK
Although cooking is done primarily with the use of heat or fire, microwaving is a modern cooking process that is gaining global popularity. Microwaves use waves of energy that cause molecules to vibrate, build heat and cook the food. As less – or no – water can be used when cooking items such as vegetables, if not overcooked, microwave cooking can help preserve some nutrients.

The nutrients lost during cooking varies depending on the food and the way in which it is cooked.

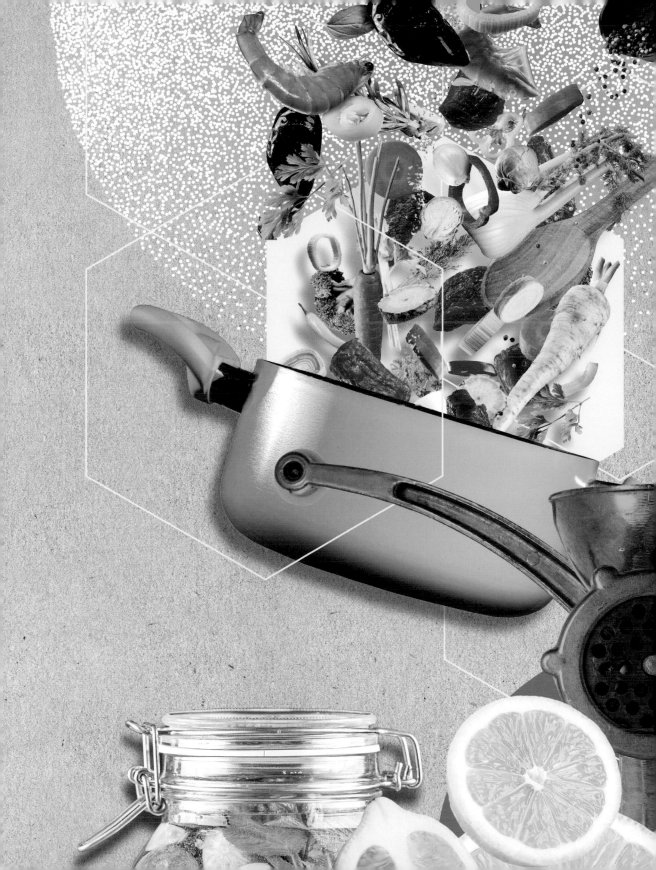

REFINING

the 30-second digest

Refined foods are processed or altered so that they are no longer in their natural state, a process that results in a loss of beneficial nutrients and fibre. A whole grain contains an endosperm, germ and bran – all nutrients remain intact. Automated milling using a roller mill is used as a process to create refined grains, producing a finer texture and extending shelf life. This processing method improves the digestibility of nutrients embedded within the grain; however, it strips the bran and germ from the grain to leave the endosperm – the nutrients are no longer intact. A refined grain is missing several B vitamins, iron and dietary fibre, and numerous other nutrients are reduced. The refined process occurs in foods beyond grains, commonly in sugars and oils. These products lack nutrients and minerals as compared to their wholesome counterparts. Foods that contain refined products (white sugar, white flour, oils) include baked goods, confectionary and processed foods. A process called 'enrichment' can reintroduce nutrients, to improve the nutritional quality of refined products. Refined foods can be overeaten due to a poorer satiety index and, due to their lack of nutrition density, should be replaced with whole foods that maximize nutritional value.

3-SECOND BITE
Refined foods are highly processed grains, sugars and oils that are stripped of a majority of their nutrients.

3-MINUTE SNACK
Refining grains were initially created for two reasons: to enhance efficiency of grain processing; to reduce rancidity of grain flour for travellers during long migrations. This process, now semi-counterbalanced with enrichment, produces a less nutritious grain product. It is advantageous for consumers to replace refined foods with whole foods, to enhance the nutritional quality of the foods they eat.

RELATED TOPICS
See also
GRAINS & GLUTEN
page 64

SALT & BLOOD PRESSURE
page 104

SUGARS & SUGAR
SUBSTITUTES
page 106

3-SECOND BIOGRAPHIES
OLIVER EVANS
1755–1819
American inventor who developed the first automated flour mill, to make grain processing more efficient without the assistance of manual labour.

JOHN STEVENS
1840–1920
English inventor who developed the roller mill, widely used today, to extract a grain's endosperm.

30-SECOND TEXT
Kristen Hicks-Roof

Replacing refined white rice and pasta with their 'whole' grain counterpart will confer many health benefits.

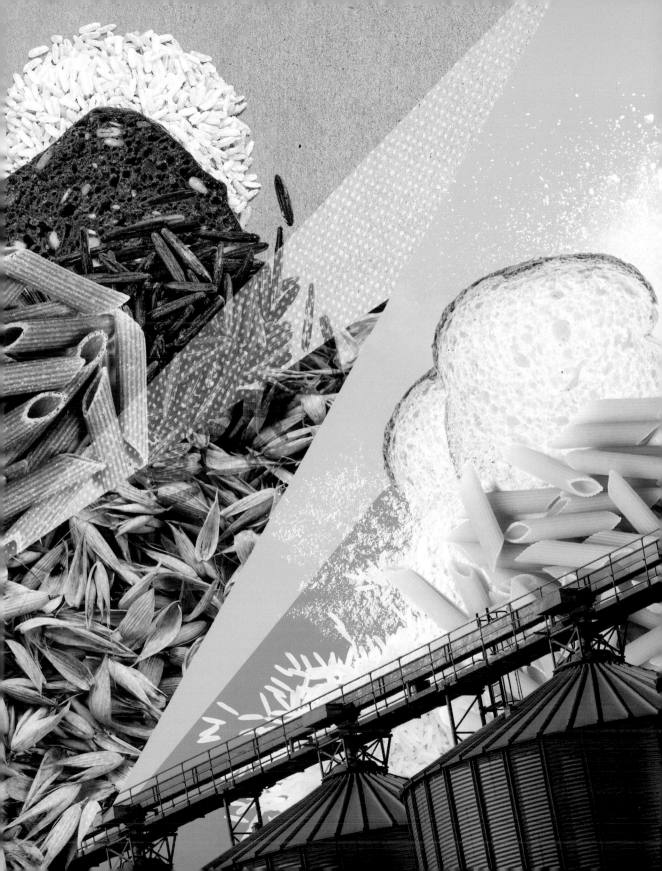

ADDITIVES

the 30-second digest

Usually when discussing
additives we are talking about components added intentionally to a food to affect its characteristic. The purpose of intentional additives is to improve the look or appeal of a food by modifying its flavour, colour, smell or texture, increasing its storage life, protecting or increasing its nutrients, or improving performance. There are many classes of additives, such as: preservatives, sweeteners, colouring agents, flavours and spices, flavour enhancers, fat replacers, nutrients, emulsifiers, thickeners, stabilizers, texturizers, binders, acid or alkalinity control agents, leaveners, anti-caking agents, humectants, yeast nutrients, dough conditioners or straighteners, firming agents, enzymes and gases. Some additives may provide more than one function; for example, ascorbic acid is a nutrient that also acts as a preservative, antioxidant or colour stabilizer. The most common additives are sugar, salt, corn syrup, citric acid, baking soda, mustard, pepper and colouring agents made from vegetables. Countries have their own lists of permitted additives and review these lists periodically. Additives do not pose a risk to health. However, they can become an issue if someone with a sensitivity to a particular additive consumes them or if they are overconsumed.

3-SECOND BITE
Intentional additives are components added to foods for a variety of reasons and functions, such as to enhance flavour or as a fat replacement.

3-MINUTE SNACK
Use of additives is controversial. Some believe they should not be used at all and others believe they are appropriate to use. While some additives' functions are not considered essential and, therefore, should be disallowed (such as colouring agents), some additives provide functions that are beneficial to a product (such as preservation, so you can keep your bread for a week instead of a couple of days before it goes stale).

RELATED TOPICS
See also
FOOD ALLERGIES
& INTOLERANCES
page 100

COOKING, PROCESSING
& PRESERVING
page 134

LABELS & PACKAGING
page 140

3-SECOND BIOGRAPHY
FREDERICK (OR FRIEDRICH)
ACCUM
1769–1838
German chemist who published *Treatise on Adulteration of Food*, in which he denounced the use of chemical additives to food, causing considerable friction with food processors and manufacturers.

30-SECOND TEXT
Judith Rodriguez

It has been suggested that some additives may cause hyperactivity and behavioural problems in children.

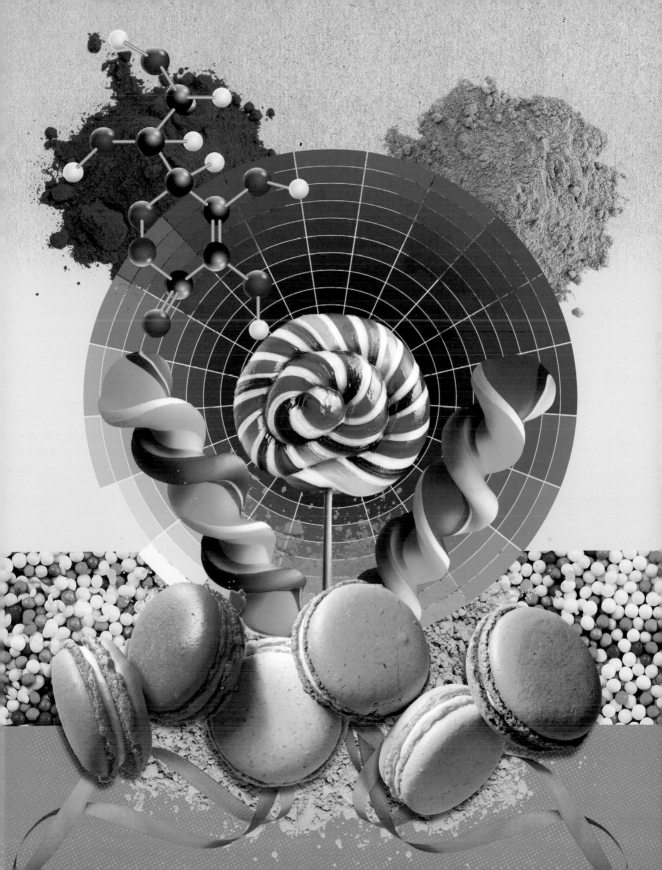

LABELS & PACKAGING

the 30-second digest

Modern food packaging has its
roots in the Napoleonic Wars (1803–15), when
the French government offered a 12,000-franc
reward for the invention of a method of
providing transportable, stable and safe food to
soldiers in the field, which lead to the invention
of food canning. Technological advances have
allowed for the majority of foodstuffs to be
purchased pre-packaged. Nowadays, packaging
protects food from the point it is processed to
when it is purchased by the consumer, whilst
maintaining the product's nutritional and
sensory qualities. Packaging also provides
product details, including a list of ingredients
with allergens and additives identified, the
'best before' or 'use by' date and nutritional
information. The World Health Organization
(WHO) advises that nutritional labelling of
pre-packaged foods should be in line with
international standards, including the *Codex
Alimentarius* – a 'food code' that ensures
consumer protection and fair trade. Since
December 2016, back-of-pack labelling has
become a mandatory requirement of pre-
packaged foods, under EU legislation. The
WHO European Food and Nutrition Action
Plan 2015–20 calls for countries to develop
and implement front-of-pack labelling systems
for consumer-friendly nutritional information.

RELATED TOPICS
See also
SALT & BLOOD PRESSURE
page 104

COOKING, PROCESSING
& PRESERVING
page 134

ADDITIVES
page 138

3-SECOND BITE
Nutritional information on
food labels is considered
an important strategy for
encouraging consumers to
make informed and healthy
diet choices.

3-MINUTE SNACK
Saturated fat, sugar and
salt-rich processed foods
are major contributors
to the global burden of
chronic diseases. It is vital
to provide consumers with
accurate and easy-to-
understand nutritional
food labels, in line with
government dietary
recommendations. Further
research is needed to
examine links between
nutrition knowledge,
food label usage and
food intake; this will aid
the development of
educational programmes
that promote healthier diet
choices in less informed
and/or educated consumer
groups.

3-SECOND BIOGRAPHIES
NICOLAS APPERT
1749–1841
French chef, confectioner and
distiller, who was also known
as the 'father of canning' for
his pioneering work on airtight
food preservation.

ERIK WALLENBERG
1915–99
Swedish engineer who was
responsible for inventing the
Tetra Pak tetrahedron-shaped
milk package.

30-SECOND TEXT
Oonagh Markey

*Nutrient profiling
systems, such as the
traffic light colour-
coding system, are
increasingly popular.*

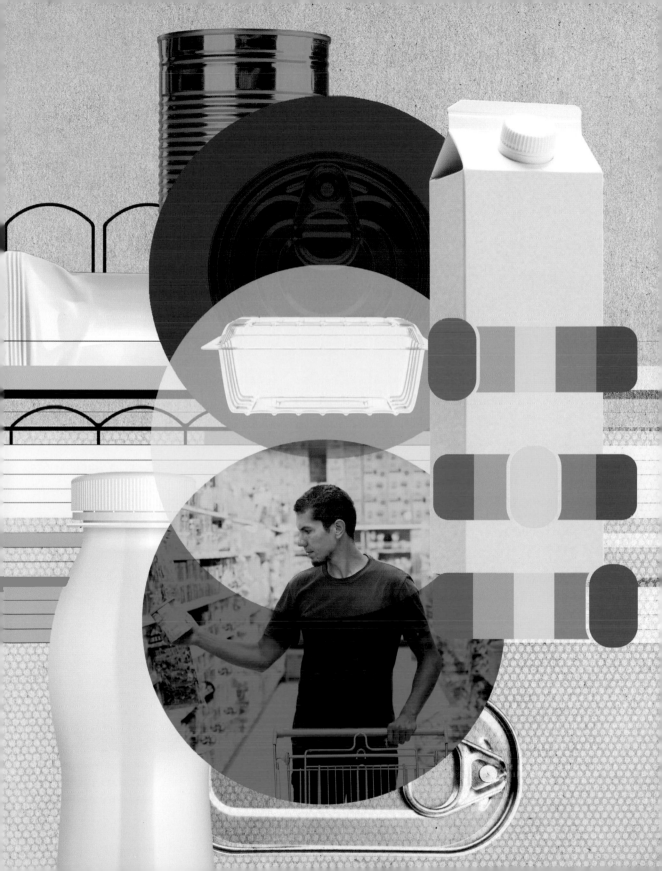

ORGANIC FOODS

the 30-second digest

The demand for organic foods

has increased, particularly in developed countries. The motivation for choosing to buy organic food varies, but includes the beliefs that it is less environmentally damaging, contains no chemical residues and is associated with better animal welfare than conventionally produced foods. Scientific reviews have reported that organic food crops can have higher antioxidant activity than conventional crops, which also contain more nitrate, the consumption of which has been associated with both good and negative effects on health. There is also evidence that organic milk and meat contain higher amounts of omega-3 polyunsaturated fats than conventional counterparts, but whilst the percentage increase often appears significant, since normal foods contain very little of these fats, the higher values in the organic products are not likely to impact the diet as a whole. There is evidence that organic milk contains less of some important nutrients, notably iodine and selenium, than conventional milk, which could contribute to an already worryingly low intake of these nutrients in some sections of the population. Overall, there is little or no evidence that long-term consumption of organic foods will lower the risk of nutrition-related ill health than eating conventional foods.

3-SECOND BITE
The classification of organic food varies country to country, but generally the focus is on environmentally-conscious farming, without the use of synthetic pesticides or fertilizers.

3-MINUTE SNACK
Before World War II, foods from crops and animals were all organic, but not labelled so. In the 1940s, an organic movement began due to worries about the increasing use of chemical fertilizers and pesticides in increasingly industrialized agricultural practices. Largely as a result of environmental awareness, popularity grew, and standardized certification procedures followed. Today, some governments support organic farming through agricultural subsidy reform.

RELATED TOPICS
See also
DIETARY FATS & HEART DISEASE
page 98

NITRATE & NITRITE
page 118

FREE-RANGE & INTENSIVELY FARMED FOODS
page 144

3-SECOND BIOGRAPHIES
WALTER JAMES
1896–1982
British agriculturalist who created the term 'organic farming' and is regarded as the 'father' of modern organic agriculture.

LADY EVELYN BALFOUR
1898–1990
British organic farming pioneer who graduated in 1918 with a diploma in agriculture from what is now the University of Reading. Founded the Soil Association in 1946.

30-SECOND TEXT
Ian Givens

Organic cows enjoy a diet free from artificial additives, chemicals and GM ingredients.

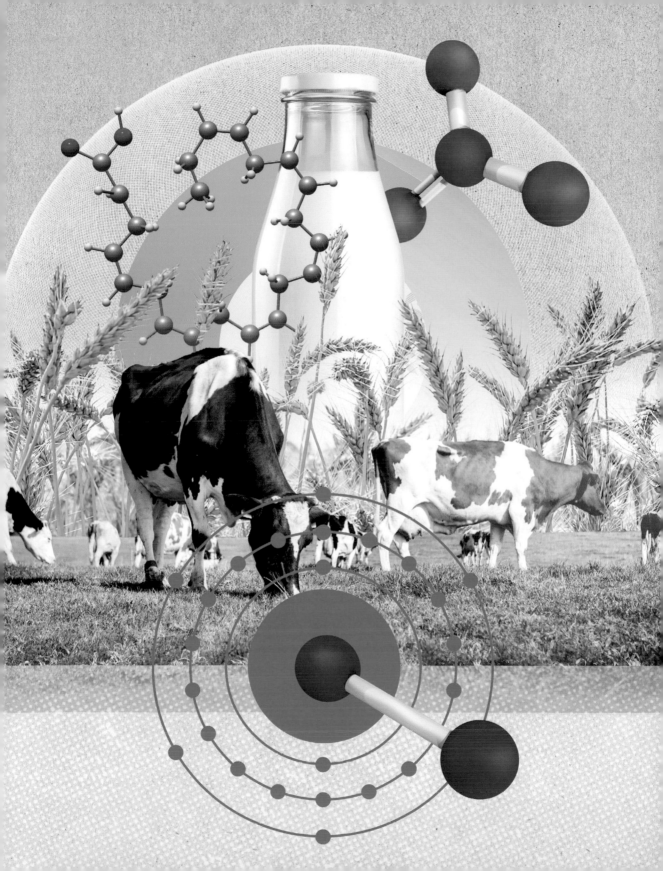

FREE-RANGE & INTENSIVELY FARMED FOODS

the 30-second digest

Intensification of animal

production began in the 1950s to increase food production. This involved more animals being kept indoors, particularly meat poultry, hens and pigs that have diets based on cereals. There followed some increased housing of beef cattle and dairy cows, and some supermarkets now demand that dairy cows have to graze outdoors for a certain period per year. There has been increased demand for foods from animals in free-range systems, likely due to perceived higher animal welfare and ethics of production. Whether foods produced by animals in free-range systems are nutritionally superior to those produced from intensive systems has many similarities to the organic versus non-organic foods debate. As with organic foods, beef, lamb and milk from outdoor grazing cattle have been shown to contain somewhat higher amounts of omega-3 polyunsaturated fats than those from animals kept indoors. There is also similar evidence for free-range poultry meat, and eggs from free-range hens have been shown to have a higher vitamin D content than those that are battery farmed. However, milk from grazing cows is likely to contain less iodine and selenium than from animals fed diets to which these nutrients are added.

RELATED TOPICS
See also
DIETARY FATS &
HEART DISEASE
page 98

ORGANIC FOODS
page 142

3-SECOND BIOGRAPHIES
HIPPOCRATES OF KOS
c. 460–c. 370 BCE
An influential Greek physician who also considered food ethics, advising that, 'Food products yielded by nature have to be improved and refined.'

KARL MARX
1818–83
German revolutionary socialist who considered the ethics of food production, saying that, 'The food products generated by capitalism represent a basic experience of estrangement and alienation.'

30-SECOND TEXT
Ian Givens

3-SECOND BITE
Currently – and perhaps surprisingly – there is no clear evidence that foods from free-range animals are of superior nutritional quality than those produced more intensively.

3-MINUTE SNACK
So-called 'ethical omnivorism' is a philosophy and a diet that makes it essential only to consume foods that come from animals that are grass fed and free range. Similarly, only wild fish caught ethically and sustainably farmed fish can be consumed. One aim is to ensure that animals are managed and slaughtered according to ethical principles, with the hope that more retailers and restaurants will give consumers the choice.

Overall, no evidence yet exists that free-range produced foods are healthier than those from intensive systems.

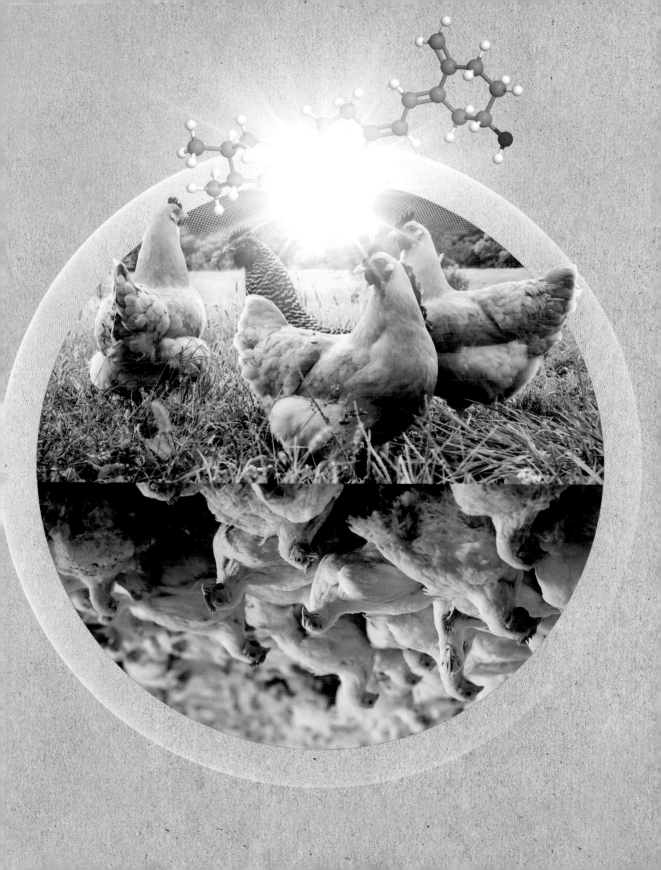

GM FOODS

the 30-second digest

Genetically modified (GM)

organisms are those whose genetic material (DNA) has been altered in a way that doesn't occur naturally through reproduction. Scientists introduce a new gene from a different organism, even one unrelated to the modified species. DNA can be taken from plants, invertebrates or bacteria and inserted into the target species. The main purpose is to enhance plant yield and improve resistance to pests and diseases, but some DNA crosses have resulted in strange outcomes, such as glow in the dark mice. Examples of GM food applications include corn, oilseed rape, sugar beet and soya, as well as less allergenic milk from cows that have been engineered to express lower levels of beta-lactoglobulin. Regulation differs depending on the country, and even if GM foods are not grown commercially, certain crops, such as maize, soybean and sugar beet, might be imported. Concerns about GM organisms include the potential for them to escape and spread to wild populations, unintended consequences for other species of animals or insects, loss of biodiversity, increased use of pesticides, heightened allergenicity and safety of GM foods. WHO has stated that GM foods need to be assessed on a case-by-case basis.

RELATED TOPICS
See also
NUTRIENT–GENE
INTERACTIONS
page 42

FOOD ALLERGIES
& INTOLERANCES
page 102

FOOD SUSTAINABILITY
page 148

3-SECOND BIOGRAPHIES
GREGOR MENDEL
1822–84
Augustinian friar and scientist considered to be the founder of genetics, thanks to his meticulous research in breeding different characteristics in pea plants.

HUGO DE VRIES
1848–1935
Dutch botanist who postulated that the inheritance of specific traits was due to hereditary carriers called 'pangenes', shortened later to 'genes'.

30-SECOND TEXT
Carrie Ruxton

WHO has stated that all GM foods currently on the market for human consumption are safe.

3-SECOND BITE
Genetically modified foods provide benefits to food producers and sometimes consumers, but acceptability has remained low in many developed countries.

3-MINUTE SNACK
Farmers have been genetically modifying plants and animals for hundreds of years by selective breeding. GM took this up a level by enabling a wider genepool – even across different species – as well as shortening the time to create a desired characteristic. Depending upon your viewpoint, the potential of GM could be positive, heralding an era of cheap nutritious ingredients, or negative, raising the possibility of 'Frankenstein' or unsafe foods.

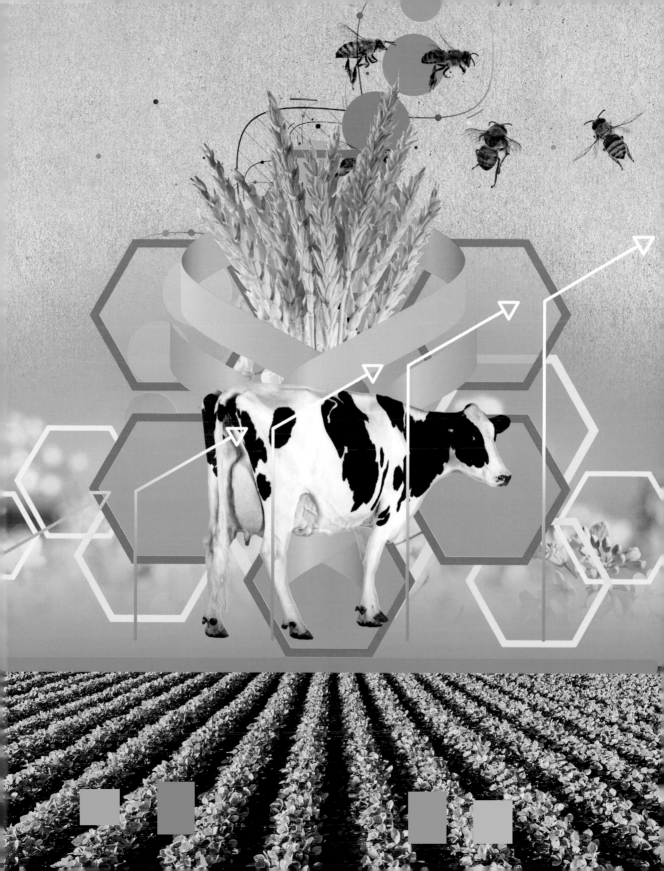

FOOD SUSTAINABILITY

the 30-second digest

The term 'sustainability' refers to using a resource without depleting or damaging the resource. There are five elements considered important in sustainable agriculture, all of which relate to food sustainability: water quality and supply; animal and plant biodiversity; energy production and use; plant and animal production; labour practices (as they relate to social justice and equity). Sustainability, including food sustainability, is guided by the underlying philosophy that as 'stewards' of the Earth, we have a responsibility to care for it and benefit from its abundant resources, but not deplete or destroy them in the process. This may also guide some persons to emphasize, focus on or select specific types of diets or food-related behaviours, such as vegetarianism or eating only organic or free-trade foods. There are different types of farming and scales (sizes of farms). Whilst there is an assumption that small farms promote food sustainability and large farms (agribusiness) does not, the type of process, efficiency and impact on ecology and labourers should be the determinant of the sustainability of the practice. There is controversy concerning the sustainability and impact of genetic engineering. Nevertheless, focus on a plant-based diet is generally regarded as being more eco-friendly than an omnivorous diet.

RELATED TOPICS
See also
VEGAN & VEGETARIANISM
page 66

ORGANIC FOODS
page 142

GM FOODS
page 146

3-SECOND BIOGRAPHIES
MASANOBU FUKUOKA
1913–2008
Japanese farmer, philosopher and author of the bestselling *The One-Straw Revolution*; a leader in the worldwide sustainable agriculture movement.

WENDELL BERRY
1934–
Renowned American sustainable food pioneer, author and activist.

30-SECOND TEXT
Judith Rodriguez

Biodynamic farms are managed as self-sustaining whole organisms, with everything in balance.

3-SECOND BITE
Food sustainability can be promoted by emphasizing a diet with plant-based foods, shopping local and using recyclable bags, while minimizing the use of plastics, excessive packaging and food waste.

3-MINUTE SNACK
The Great Law of the Iroquois (Native American) Confederacy stated that deliberations must consider the impact on the seventh generation, approximately 150 years into the future. That has become a basic principle underlying the concept of sustainability – often referred to as 'Seventh Generation Sustainability'. This philosophy is not unique to the Iroquois; many nations, tribes and indigenous people around the world live by it.

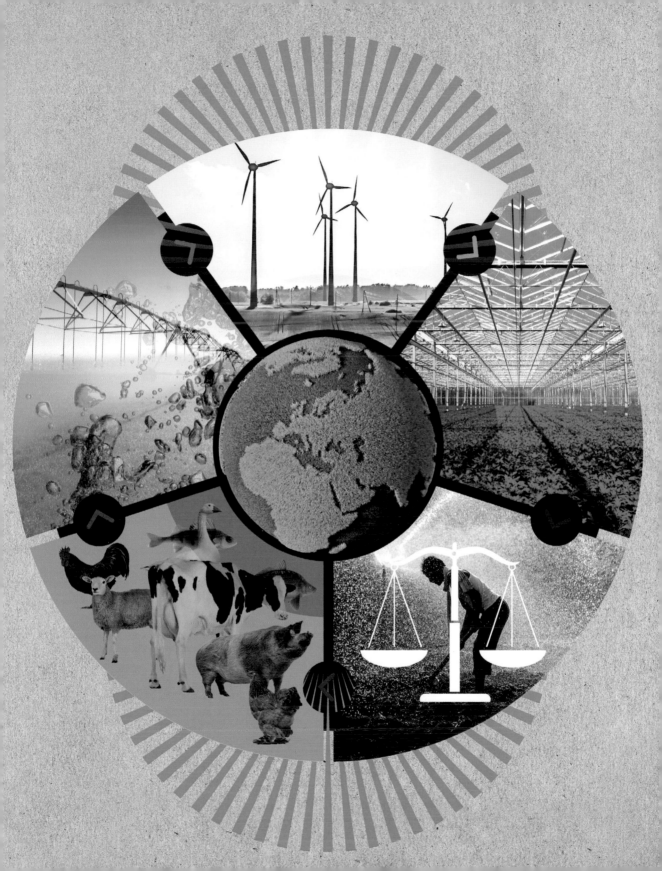

22 October 1896
Born in Entiat, Washington, USA

1918
Attends Washington State College, but studies are interrupted by WWI, during which time King serves with the 12th Infantry Machine Gun Company

1919
Marries Hilda Bainton, with whom he has one daughter and two sons

1923
Graduates from the University of Pittsburgh with an MSc and then a PhD

1931–32
Isolates vitamin C crystals from lemon juice and, using an animal model, identifies these as the cure for scurvy

1942
Becomes first Scientific Director of the Nutrition Foundation

1950–53
President of the International Union of Nutrition Sciences (IUNS)

1951
Elected to the National Academy of Sciences

1962
Retires from teaching and becomes a consultant to the Rockefeller Foundation

23 January 1988
Dies in Pennsylvania, USA

CHARLES GLEN KING

Although the Nobel Prize in 1937 for the discovery of vitamin C was awarded to Hungarian scientist Albert Szent-Györgyi, many believed that the honour should have been shared with Charles Glen King, an American pioneer of vitamin research.

Known to his friends as Glen, King was born in 1896 on a homestead near a small town in Washington State. Having only a rudimentary local school, King was spurred on to attend university a year early, where he chose to pursue studies in Geology before switching to Chemistry. Emerging later than usual from his undergraduate studies, due to the onset of World War I, King moved to Pittsburgh University. There, he enrolled in a Masters degree in Chemistry before beginning a PhD in Organic Chemistry. During this time, he married Hilda Bainton and settled in the Pittsburgh area to raise their children, making sure that the babies were given fresh orange juice daily, even though he was yet to isolate the active ingredient, vitamin C.

It was already known by 1922 that citrus fruits contained a vital component that could ward off scurvy, a serious condition characterized by weakness, joint pains, bleeding gums and blood spots, which typically affected sailors on long voyages. Scientists were desperate to understand exactly which chemical in citrus was responsible for the health benefits, leading to a global, yet unconnected, research effort.

Working in laboratories in Hungary and England, Szent-Györgyi detected an antioxidant compound in adrenal samples, which he named 'hexuronic acid' in 1927. What he didn't know at the time was that he was looking at vitamin C. On the other side of the Atlantic, King and his team were trying to isolate the anti-scurvy factor from lemon juice using meticulous animal feeding experiments. By April 1932, they were able to publish a report in *Science* describing the isolation of the vitamin C crystal and, later that year, its chemical structure. However, a rival paper by Szent-Györgyi was published two weeks later, confirming that hexuronic acid and vitamin C were one and the same.

The awarding of the Nobel Prize to Szent-Györgyi in 1937 for his work in discovering vitamin C was a disappointment to King. While Szent-Györgyi was the first to note the existence of hexuronic acid, there is doubt that he understood its biological significance until King's research had been completed.

Carrie Ruxton

APPENDICES

RESOURCES

NUTRITION WEBSITES

British Nutrition Foundation (BNF)
www.nutrition.org.uk
Impartial, evidence-based information
on food and nutrition.

European Food Information Council (Eufic)
www.eufic.org
A non-profit organization that offers science-
based information on food and health.

Nutrition Society
www.nutritionsociety.org
Advances the scientific study of nutrition
and its application to health.

Eatwell Guide UK
www.gov.uk/government/publications/
the-eatwell-guide
A policy tool used to define government
recommendations on eating healthily and
achieving a balanced diet.

Association for Nutrition (AfN)
www.associationfornutrition.org
Independent regulator for registered
nutritionists.

British Dietetic Association (BDA)
www.bda.uk.com/foodfacts/home
The only body in the UK representing
the whole of the dietetic workforce.

Scientific Advisory Committee on Nutrition
www.gov.uk/government/groups/scientific-
advisory-committee-on-nutrition
Advises Public Health England on nutrition and
related health matters.

Public Health England (PHE)
www.gov.uk/government/organisations/
public-health-england
Aims to protect and improve the nation's health
and well-being, and reduce health inequalities.

Institute of Food Science and Technology (IFST)
www.ifst.org
Leading professional body for those involved in
all aspects of food science and technology.

Nutrition.gov
www.nutrition.gov
Information to make healthy eating choices.

Academy of Nutrition and Dietetics
www.eatright.org
Science-based food and nutrition information,
a consumer site from the Academy.

United States Department of Agriculture
(USDA) Agricultural Research Service
ndb.nal.usda.gov/ndb
Food Composition databases.

Nutrition Source
www.hsph.harvard.edu/nutritionsource
Harvard Public Health site for evidence-based
diet and nutrition information.

Consumer Lab
www.consumerlab.com
Test results and information to help
consumers and healthcare professionals
evaluate related products.

Center for Science in the Public Interest
cspinet.org
Advice for a healthier food system.

Canadian Nutrition Society/Société
Canadienne de Nutrition (CNS/SCN)
cns-scn.ca
Provides all sectors with an interest
in nutrition access to evidence-based
information, resources and expertise.

Nutrition Australia
www.nutritionaustralia.org
An independent, member organization
that promotes health and well-being.

The Nutrition Society of Australia (NSA)
nsa.asn.au
Scientists and educators who aim to increase
and communicate the scientific value and
relevance of nutrition science in Australia.

The Nutrition Society of New Zealand
www.nutritionsociety.ac.nz
Promotes the science of nutrition and its role
in growth and development, health and well-
being in humans and animals.

HEALTH/MEDICAL WEBSITES
World Health Organization (WHO)
www.who.int
Includes publications, a Health Topics directory
and Global Health Observatory (GHO) data.

The BMJ
www.bmj.com
Host to research, education, news and views,
and campaigns information.

NHS
www.nhs.uk/conditions
Up-to-date and easy to understand directory of
illness and disease.

WebMD
www.webmd.com
Health and medical news and information.

Medline Plus
medlineplus.gov/nutrition.html
US National Institute of Health's National
Library of Medicine website, for consumers.

NOTES ON CONTRIBUTORS

EDITOR

Julie A Lovegrove is Professor of Human Nutrition and Director of the Hugh Sinclair Unit of Human Nutrition at the University of Reading, and a Registered Nutritionist. Her expertise is nutritional influences on cardiometabolic risk, including nutrient-gene interactions.

CONTRIBUTORS

Margaret Ashwell OBE was Senior Research Scientist with the Medical Research Council, Principal of the Good Housekeeping Institute and Science Director of the British Nutrition Foundation. She became President of the Association for Nutrition in 2016.

Luke Bell is a Plant Biologist, Food Chemist and Nutritional Science Researcher from the University of Reading.

Jenna Braddock is a Certified Specialist in Sports Dietetics and works primarily with adolescent athletes. She is faculty at the University of North Florida, writes at MakeHealthyEasy.com and works with teen athletes and their parents.

Philip C Calder is Professor of Nutritional Immunology within Medicine at the University of Southampton. His work aims to understand how nutrition affects the functioning of the human body.

Rosalind Fallaize is a Registered Dietitian and Research Fellow in Nutrition and Dietetics at the University of Hertfordshire and University of Reading. Her research interests include dietary assessment, eating behaviour and e-health.

Glenn Gibson is Professor of Food Microbiology and Head of Food Microbial Sciences at Reading University, and is widely regarded as the UK's leading expert in this field.

Ian Givens is Professor of Food Chain Nutrition at the University of Reading and Director of the Institute of Food, Nutrition and Health. His key interest is in human nutrition, and food chain nutrition in particular.

Bruce A Griffin is Professor of Nutritional Metabolism at the University of Surrey. He is a Biomedical Scientist with research experience in human lipid and lipoprotein metabolism, nutrition and cardiovascular disease.

Kristen Hicks-Roof is a Registered Dietitian Nutritionist and Assistant Professor at the University of North Florida. Her passion is improving the health and wellness of the everyday individual by promoting realistic dietary and lifestyle changes.

Ditte Hobbs is a Research Fellow and Registered Nutritionist at the University of Reading. Her research focuses on exploring the impact of nutrition on cardio-metabolic diseases, with interest in the effects of dietary nitrate.

Ian Macdonald is Professor at the School of Life Sciences at Nottingham University. His main interests are obesity, diabetes, nutrition and exercise physiology. He chaired the SACN Carbohydrates Working Group.

Oonagh Markey is a Vice-Chancellor's Research Fellow at Loughborough University, a Visiting Research Fellow at the University of Reading and a Registered Nutritionist. Her work aims to understand how nutrients and diet influence cardiovascular disease risk.

Elizabeth A Miles is a Nutritional Immunologist at the University of Southampton, with expertise in allergology, nutrition and dietetics and immunology.

D Joe Millward is Emeritus Professor of Human Nutrition at the University of Surrey, and has served on several international and national committees, advising on requirements for protein and food energy.

Brian Power is a Lecturer at University College London and a Registered Dietitian. His research interests include the development of behaviour change interventions.

Hilary Powers is Professor Emerita in Nutritional Biochemistry at the University of Sheffield, UK. She has worked in the area of micronutrient function for over thirty years and her work has contributed to an understanding of optimum nutrition, globally.

Judith Rodriguez is a Registered Dietitian Nutritionist, Professor at the University of North Florida. She is a Past President of the Academy of Nutrition and Dietetics. Her areas of interest include nutrition education, food and culture and health disparities.

Carrie Ruxton is a Registered Dietitian with more than 20 years' experience. Her PhD was in child nutrition and she has written more than 50 peer-reviewed publications, as well as writing for consumer and professional magazines.

Jill Snyder is a Registered Dietitian Nutritionist and Instructor at the University of North Florida, counselling clients for medical nutrition therapy and the benefits of a healthy diet, in addition to teaching at UNF.

Katherine Stephens is a Research Fellow at the University of Reading.

Jayne Woodside is Professor of Human Nutrition within the Centre for Public Health at Queen's University Belfast, where she is also Deputy Director of the Institute for Global Food Security.

Zhiping Yu, a Registered Dietitian Nutritionist and Associate Professor at the University of North Florida. Her research interests include prevention and treatment of eating disorders, obesity and obesity-related chronic diseases.

INDEX

ACKNOWLEDGEMENTS

The publisher would like to thank the following for permission to reproduce copyright material (in most cases the material has been used to create a montage):

Alamy Stock Photo/age fotostock: 90; Granger Historical Picture Archive: 30. Ancel Keys Archive, School of Public Health, University of Minnesota: 70. Hugh Sinclair Unit of Human Nutrition, University of Reading: 124; Shutterstock/29September: 117; 3d_kot: 81; 3drenderings: 37; 7 pips: 77, 147; Abramova Elena: 117, 119; adike: 59; Afanasev Ivan: 83; Africa Studio: 17, 49, 67, 77, 87, 127, 135; akepong srichaichana: 57; AlenKadr: 15, 109; Alex Mit: 127; Alexandar Iotzov: 25; Alexander Raths: 123; Alhovik: 47, 87; Alila Medical Media: 81; Alp Aksoy: 69; Amvin Mccartney: 107; anastasiia ivanova: 129; Angel Simon: 99; annarevoltosphotography: 15; Aphelleon: 127; apiguide: 105; arleksey: 41; arsa35: 87; Astronoman: 81; Asya Nurullina: 57; Avatar_023: 87; Beautyimage: 99, 135; Benkworks: 147; Bennyartist: 63; bergamont: 29, 85; Bjoern Wylezich: 25, 121; Blend Images: 83; blue-bubble: 39, 41, 65, 67, 77, 127; bonchan: 121; Borbely Edit: 39; Boule: 139; Bryan Solomon: 107; Budimir Jevtic: 85; Casther: 99; Catalin Rusnac: 43; Cecilia Lim H M: 149; Christoph Burgstedt: 43; Christos Georghiou: 147; chromatos: 15; Chutima Chaochaiya: 93; CKP1001: 107, 127; Claudio Divizia: 105; COLOA Studio: 65; conejota: 139; Coprid: 101; Creative icon styles: 23; CRS Photo: 149; Daxiao Productions: 77; Dean Drobot: 79; Decobrush: 77; deepadesigns: 67; design36: 27, 47; Diana Taliun: 49, 83, 121, 139; Digital Photo: 17; Dinozzzaver: 63; Ditty_about_summer: 141; Dmitry9131: 137; Drawbot: 89; DronG: 57, 111; Duda Vasilii: 107; Eivaisla: 111; Elena Kharichkina: 93; Elena Schweitzer: 17, 47, 81; Elena Veselova: 15; elenabsl: 89; Elgub: 137; epiximages: 77; eranicle: 27, 127; Eric Isselee: 147, 149; ermess: 23, 123; ESB Professional: 27; Eugene Onischenko: 19; EVO40: 47; Everett Historical: 59; Evgeniy Kalinovskiy: 139; Evgeny Karandaev: 29, 101; Extarz: 105; FiledImage: 61; Fokin Oleg: 25; Foxys Forest Manufacture: 69; Gen Epic Solutions: 47; gillmar: 59; giSpate: 149; Gita Kulinitch Studio: 129; Golden Faraon: 27; Golubovy: 15; grafnata: 69; grocap: 105; gst: 49; Guru 3D: 43; GzP_Design: 77; HAKKI ARSLAN: 19, 37; horiyan: 141; Hortimages: 99; Howard Sayer: 105; Hurst Photo: 87; I am Kulz: 61; ibreakstock: 27, 37, 99, 143; Ievgenii Meyer: 143; ifong: 79; Igor Dutina: 27; Igor Petrushenko: 99, 101, 105, 123; igorstevanovic: 147; Ileish Anna: 57; ilusmedical: 19; Ilya AkinsHIN: 47; Ilya Sirota: 69; Ink Drop: 123; IrenD: 143, 145; irin-k: 147; its_al_dente: 43; Ivaylo Ivanov: 139; Jacek Fulawka: 149; Jag_cz: 135; jalcaraz: 77; jeedlove: 49, 87; Jiang Hongyan: 117, 119; Jiri Hera: 93, 123; Jose Luis Calvo: 21; Juan Gaertner: 41, 61; Juan J. Jimenez: 21; Julia_Lelija: 67; kandinsky: 65, 145; Kateryna Kon: 41, 101; Kayo: 59; Kishivan: 109; KonstantinChristian: 81; Kovaleva_Ka: 65, 81, 101; kovalto1: 25; Krahovnet: 15, 25; krataechang: 107; Kriengsuk Prasroetsung: 109; kudla: 83; Kues: 15; Kundra: 149; kzww: 87; ladyfortune: 49; LanaSweet: 49; Leigh Prather: 29; Linda Bucklin: 67; LinGraphics: 141; Linnas: 19, 107, 109; Lisa S.: 137; Lisovskaya Natalia: 57; Ljupco Smokovski: 83; Lucky Business: 107; Lukas Gojda: 67; Madlen: 83, 137; Maks Narodenko: 65; Maksim Shmeljov: 85; mamanamsai: 149; MaraZe: 15, 29, 59, 111; MarcelClemens: 25; margouillat photo: 111; Marian Weyo: 135; marilyn barbone: 21, 25, 129; Marina Shanti: 111; Marius Dragne: 117; Mariyana M: 57, 79, 123; Markus Mainka: 37; MarShot: 79; Martial Red: 23; maryna rodyukova: 139; Matjoe: 63; matkub2499: 81; maximmmmum: 25; Mdesignstudio: 147; Meder Lorant: 27; Melica: 139; memej: 119; metamorworks: 41; Miceking: 123; Miloje: 79; Miroslav Cvetinov: 21; molekuul_be: 17, 21, 37, 59, 65, 81, 101, 107, 119, 123; montego: 87; Moonborne: 145; Morinka: 65; Mrs.Moon: 145; MSSA: 47; mythja: 69; naihei: 37, 143; Nataliia K: 29, 49, 121; Nattika: 85; Naypong Studio: 89; Nazzu: 121; nehophoto: 93; Nik Merkulov: 49, 67, 111, 121; Nitr: 27, 147; NY-P: 87; Ola-ola: 139; Olga Nikonova: 149; Olha Afanasieva: 57; Olhastock: 61; OliveTree: 27, 39, 61; oork: 127; ostill: 15, 39, 119, 147; OxfordSquare: 59, 83; OZaiachin: 17; Padma Inguva: 119; Paitoon Insee: 65; paul prescott: 89; Pawel Michalowski: 89; Pektoral: 117; petarg: 29; Petr Malyshev: 141; Petr Vaclavek: 85; photomaster: 149; Pi-Lens: 139; Picsfive: 93, 99; Pisuton'c: 27, 29, 121; Pormezz: 29, 67; Potapov Alexander: 121; prizma: 89; Protasov AN: 63; Pumidol: 61; Raimundo79: 17, 19, 27, 29, 117; Rawpixel.com: 49; Redshinestudio: 39; Reload Design: 25; Richard M Lee: 137; rikkyall: 39, 149; rnl: 79; Rob Bayer: 85; Roman Samokhin: 29, 57, 83, 135; Romariolen: 19; Rostislav_Sedlacek: 109; Roxana Bashyrova: 85; Rtstudio: 137; SaGa Studio: 67; sciencepics: 21; Sebastian Kaulitzki: 19, 27, 29, 43, 55, 81, 127; seeyou: 65; Sergey Bogdanov: 145; Sergey Mironov: 137; Sergiy Kuzmin: 87; sharpshutter: 69; Shawn Hempel: 27, 145; shipfactory: 93; Shutter_M: 67; sirtravelalot: 123; Slavko Sereda: 69; SosnaRadosna: 111; Spectral-Design: 129; stanislaff: 43; Stockforlife: 27, 119; Studio 1a Photography: 149; Sunny Forest: 143; Superheang168: 111; Suradech Prapairat: 61; Svetlana Lukienko: 15; symbiot: 143; T-Design: 83; Tarasyuk Igor: 109, 143; Timolina: 15, 83; Tinydevil: 101; Tonkinphotography: 63; toysf400: 23; trgrowth: 143; Undrey: 15; V O R T E X: 87; Vadarshop: 37; Valentina Razumova: 27, 61, 81, 119; Valerii Ivashchenko: 135; Valerii_Dex: 137; Valeriya_Dor: 29, 135; Vanzyst: 19, 83; Vector FX: 23, 55; Vector Tradition: 47; Vector.design: 111; VectorMine: 65; Victor Josan: 23; Vikpit: 105; Viktar Malyshchyts: 55; Vitalii Karas: 55; Vitaly Korovin: 83; vs148: 147; vvoe: 25; wavebreakmedia: 83, 109; What Photo: 109; Winston Link: 49; xpixel: 67, 83; Yakobchuk Viacheslav: 85; yaruna: 17, 105; Yarygin: 109; zcw: 81; Zenobillis: 69; zi3000: 57. University of Pittsburgh Historic Photographs, University of Pittsburgh Library System: 150. Wikimedia Commons/Doc. RNDr. Josef Reischig, CSc./CC-BY-SA-3.0: 129; Grochim/CC-BY-SA-3.0: 141; Joanna Spence/CC-BY-4.0: 102; Jynto/CC0 1.0 Universal (CC0 1.0): 121; Riccardoariotti/CC-BY-3.0: 129; Velocity2222X/CC BY-SA 3.0: 41.

All reasonable efforts have been made to trace copyright holders and to obtain their permission for the use of copyright material. The publisher apologizes for any errors or omissions in the list above and will gratefully incorporate any corrections in future reprints if notified.